Chicken Soup
for the Soul.

My
Resolution

Chicken Soup for the Soul: My Resolution
101 Stories... Great Ideas for Your Mind, Body, and...Wallet
by Jack Canfield, Mark Victor Hansen, D'ette Corona, Barbara LoMonaco

Published by Chicken Soup for the Soul Publishing, LLC   www.chickensoup.com

The publisher gratefully acknowledges the many publishers and individuals who granted Chicken Soup for the Soul permission to reprint the cited material.

Front cover photos courtesy of iStockPhoto.com/© mark wrag (wragg), and /© Robyn Mackenzie (robynmac). Back cover photo courtesy of iStockPhoto.com/©Koh Sze Kiat (Fertographer). Interior photograph courtesy of iStockPhoto.com/©christine balderas (DNY59).

Cover and Interior Design & Layout by Pneuma Books, LLC
For more info on Pneuma Books, visit www.pneumabooks.com

Distributed to the booktrade by Simon & Schuster. SAN: 200-2442

Publisher's Cataloging-in-Publication Data
(Prepared by The Donohue Group)

Chicken soup for the soul : my resolution : 101 stories-- great ideas for your
  mind, body, and-- wallet / [compiled by] Jack Canfield ... [et al.].

     p. ; cm.

  ISBN-13: 978-1-935096-28-3
  ISBN-10: 1-935096-28-1

1. Conduct of life--Literary collections. 2. Conduct of life--Anecdotes. 3. Life skills--Anecdotes. 4. Change (Psychology)--Literary collections. 5. Change (Psychology)--Anecdotes. I. Canfield, Jack, 1944- II. Title: My resolution

PN6071.C663 C45 2008
810.8/0206   2008939628

Chicken Soup for the Soul®
My Resolution

101 Stories...
Great Ideas for Your
Mind, Body, and... Wallet

Jack Canfield
Mark Victor Hansen
D'ette Corona
Barbara LoMonaco

Chicken Soup for the Soul Publishing, LLC
Cos Cob, CT

Chicken Soup for the Soul

www.chickensoup.com

Contents

❸
~A Guiding Hand~

❹
~Hello Body!~

❺
~I'm Worth It~

6
~Simple Pleasures~

7
~I Did It!~

8
~Gotta Laugh!~

❾

~With You by My Side~

❿

~Dreams Do Come True~

⓫

~I Actually Like This!~

⑫
~Coming Full Circle~

Chicken Soup for the Soul

Foreword

At one time or another, everyone has made resolutions—for New Year's, for that big birthday, at the beginning of a new month, or even on Monday! We all want to make positive changes in our lives or break the bad habits that we have acquired, so we... set goals for ourselves, make promises to change, pledge to improve, or make to-do lists. It doesn't matter when you start or what you call it, everyone makes commitments to improve. Resolutions can be life changing or really quite simple. Whether big or small, they will affect your entire life.

We found that some of the most popular resolutions people make are: to spend more time with family and friends; exercise and eat right; lose weight; quit smoking; make amends or reestablish a relationship; go green; go back to school; help others; get organized; downsize and simplify our lives and our finances.

After reading the thousands of stories that people submitted, one thing became very clear. Resolutions are pretty easy to make but they are not easy to keep. Change is not easy to achieve. We found that many people made the same resolutions time after time. Does that mean that the resolutions they made were not realistic? After making resolutions, some people came to the realization that they didn't really need to change; they are fine just the way they are. Some people realized that more was not always better; a bigger house or a faster car wasn't really the answer. Sometimes less rather than more was the solution.

This book is the first step in setting aside some time to take a look at your life. Like some of our contributors, you might decide that you are fine just the way you are! You are in charge of your life. You can make any changes that you want, or you can resolve to be satisfied and happy with what you already have. Whichever is the case, we hope that the stories in this book will make you think, make you laugh, make you cry, make you say "ahhh" and touch your heart as they did ours.

~Barbara LoMonaco and D'ette Corona

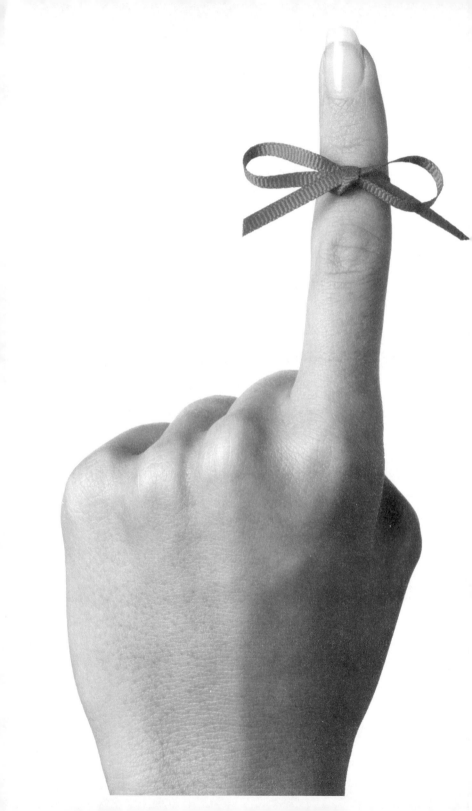

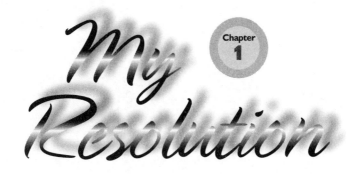

Chapter
1

From This Day Forward

It takes courage to grow up and become who you really are.

~e.e. cummings

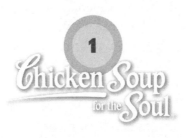

Two Little Words with a Big Impact

Too many people miss the silver lining because they're expecting gold.
~Maurice Setter

have always considered myself a positive thinker, an upbeat person and an optimist. I try to find the best in every situation. I've recently become aware of how two little words in my vocabulary have had a tremendous impact on people. I didn't even realize it.

I've been listening to myself lately, and I don't like the way I sound. As a veteran teacher, I know that praise can be a huge motivational tool. I realize the importance of developing a child's self-esteem. I generously sprinkle uplifting comments around my classroom like I am fertilizing flowers. Each new school year brings a garden variety of students, and they all blossom with praise and encouragement. I know how to thank my grown kids, my grandkids and my husband for a job well done. I toss compliments to the unsuspecting if it appears someone needs a lift. I also yo-yo my positive comments right back when I use the word that makes my preschoolers giggle—BUT.

When one of my students attempted to print her name, I oohed and ahhed. "Wow! That is a great A, and your letter, D is nice and tall, but your letter, E should be short; can you erase it and try to make it shorter?" I asked. She wasn't crushed by my comment. She tried to live up to my expectation. I thought I was helping, preparing her for kindergarten, showing her the difference in size between upper case and lower case letters. I don't believe that my comment would have any long term affect on her self-worth. I imagine though, if I'd substituted the word BUT with the word AND, she'd have been proud of her accomplishment instead of questioning the "right way" to print her name. I wish I had said, "I like your nice tall letters, AND I like how hard you are trying to make your letter E."

My recently divorced daughter called to tell me about a house she was interested in. I listened to her. I applauded her for moving forward with her life, and I said, "Honey, I am glad that you've found something you like, but...." There, I did it again! "Don't you think, with the gas prices, you might want to buy closer to your work?" As she told me all about the prospective house, I could hear the excitement and joy in her voice. The moment I spoke the word, BUT, it was as if I pricked a balloon with a needle. I could hear her slowly deflate. I sure wish I'd used the word AND. "Honey, I'm glad you found a house in your price range, AND I'm happy for you." She knows I freely express my opinions, and I know she's used to my mouth. I suspect that if I had leashed my tongue, her emotions wouldn't have flip-flopped, and we'd have both hung up feeling better.

Recently I visited my son and his six-year-old little boy and six-month-old daughter. I scooped up my grandchildren and bragged. He babysits while my daughter-in-law works weekends. I told him he was a great father; I praised him for his devotion to his family. He beamed as though he was a little boy, and then I flubbed. "You should be commended for spending your whole day taking your little boy to his sports events, but don't you think he might be worn out and ready for a bath?" There I was with my bad word again! My son's smile slid away, and he said, "He'll be fine. I'll get him to bed soon." I planted an ounce of doubt, when I should have been planting the seeds of confidence. I wish I'd said, "You're a good father, AND I admire your ability to recognize the children's individual needs."

My granddaughter showed up at my door dressed like a princess on her way to the prom. I told her how beautiful she looked. I told her I was proud of the young lady she has become, and I said, "Sweetheart,

I want you to have a great time, but please don't drink tonight." I know she doesn't engage in risky behavior; she's responsible and sensible and trustworthy. She looked as though I'd snatched her crown. "Nana!" The tone of her voice indicated how I'd made her feel. How I wish I'd said, "I want you to have a great time, AND I trust you."

My dear husband helps around the house; he did the dishes, emptied the dishwasher, and folded the laundry. I was thrilled he had lightened my work load. I thanked him. I told him how wonderful he is, and I used that naughty word again. "BUT, why did you leave crumbs all over the counter?" Why? Why? Why didn't I say, "Thank you, AND I appreciate all you do around the house."

I've been doing some self-reflecting. I've given up on losing those twenty pounds. I've decided a walk around the neighborhood is a good substitute for vigorous exercise. I've watched dust bunnies cuddle under the sofa. I've prayed in the dark instead of at church more often than not. In other words, all those New Year's resolutions are now null and void. I lose a pound; I eat a chocolate; I gain a pound. The bar on my treadmill makes a nice rack for hanging laundry. I've attended church for grandchildren's christenings, and I pass the sanctuary on my way to the church office. I vacuum on weekends. I figure if the dust bunnies don't mind snuggling for another day, I don't care either.

My house isn't spotless, my thighs are heavy, my soul, like my face could use some uplifting, but I have decided that I simply cannot keep all those resolutions I made on January 1st. I'm ready for some spring cleaning. I'm tossing those old resolutions out and I am making one, just one, which I intend to keep. I am going to refrain from using the B word. I think I can do it, and I am going to give it my best. I know it will have a positive effect on others. BUT if I mess up, I will try again, and again, and again to remove that naughty little word from my vocabulary. I resolve to replace it with the word AND. This is a resolution I intend to keep!

~Linda O'Connell

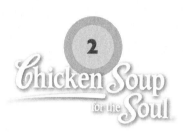

Let's Face It

A smile is an inexpensive way to change your looks.
~Charles Gordy

"What a crabby-looking lady," the cashier at my local convenience store whispered to her co-worker. I was tromping through the toilet paper aisle grabbing products off the shelf like it was Y2K all over again. I had a half dozen kids waiting for me in the van, and here's the thing: they were all my own children. No time for polite. No casual conversation with the checkout lady, no nod of approval toward the stock boy, no breathing. Just get the toilet paper, two gallons of milk and some Frosted Flakes and get back out in the trenches!

But I was intrigued by the crabby-looking lady. Which one was she? Hoisting a family pack of toilet paper under my arm, I scanned the tiny store for the crabby lady. Let's see, there's a middle-aged guy in aisle three stocking up on pork rinds, an older gentleman at the checkout purchasing an egg salad sandwich and a coffee, and... just then I saw her, the crabby-looking lady.

Her eyes were small slits; her brown hair was pulled back in a ponytail so tight it looked like her forehead would snap off. Her mouth was a severe gash between pinched cheeks. A deep furrow cut the lady's brows. Crabby wasn't the word. This lady looked like she had either smelled something really bad or was about to single-handedly euthanize her own cat. Couldn't tell which. Then, I turned away from my own reflection in the convex security mirror at the back of the store. The crabby looking lady... was me!

That night, after I ran the troops through bath, brush and bed routine, I plopped on my bed and sobbed. I was the crabby-looking lady! Me! The girl voted nicest smile by her high school class. I had become a cross between Morticia from *The Addams Family* and a lemon! Right then and there I resolved to do one thing over the next year. One simple resolution: to smile. I didn't need to wait for January 1st—I would start right now. Simple, right? Sure, if you're a televangelist. Or naturally nice. Or just had a lobotomy. But I'm a mom. And moms have stuff to accomplish. People depend on us to be crabby! How else do bedrooms get picked up?

I mean, a smile is perfectly appropriate for those "Oh, sweetie, thanks for picking a handful of dandelions for mommy and saying you wuv wuv wuv me" days. But what about the days when the teenagers broke curfew and the dog puked Oreos on the bathroom floor and Dad is late from work again and the baby is doing that colicky thing? On days like that I'm just supposed to (twitch, twitch) smile?

Well, unless I wanted to end up looking like a shrunken head, all I could do was try. Of course I didn't tell anyone about my smile resolution. I mean, it was going to be hard enough to smile without my kids making comments like, "Mom, is there something wrong with your face?" I would just go smiley on my own terms. At least ten times a day, I would make a conscious effort to smile. And it wouldn't count if I did it ten times in a row. It had to be... incremental.

The first day of "Mission Smile" I smiled at (and this is in order): a strange dog who peed on my daughter's new school shoes (while she was in them), the mailman, three of my six children (I couldn't muster more than a smirk for the teenagers just yet), a librarian who asked me if I was aware of the global overpopulation problem, and my bathtub. I smiled at my husband over the phone when he called to say he'd be late from work (it wasn't really much of a smile, more like a facial spasm). And I smiled at myself in the mirror twice, just to remind myself what a smile looked like. (Mouth curved upwards, twinkle in eyes, good... now think happy thoughts.)

After the first week of smiling practice, I discovered that if I forgot to smile all morning, I could make up for it by watching *I Love Lucy* reruns after the kids went to bed. I thought of it as extra credit smiling homework.

After a month, though, a weird thing happened. I didn't even try to find things to smile at and I'd still notice this funny sensation take over my face. It was like Pavlov's dogs to a bell: I'd see my kids run in from playing "throw mud at the sibling with the lowest IQ" and Ding! Smile. When my teenage daughter loaded the dishwasher with her soccer shin pads and cleats... Ding! Smile. Even when we were really late for church and fangs began to protrude from my upper jaw and venom dripped from my incisors and I hissed, "Hurry little children, it's time to partake in the precious body and blood of Christ!" Ding! Smile. It was actually kind of unsettling, this smile thing. Like I could actually be happy in the midst of chaos!

The final blow came, though, after nine months or so of my resolution. I was meeting a couple of friends for our regular date at a local coffee shop. Bursting though the coffee shop door in my usual haphazard manner, I overheard the cashier behind the coffee counter remark to a co-worker, "There's that happy looking lady again."

And I didn't even have to look around the coffee shop to know who she was talking about. I could see my own reflection in the cash register on the counter. The forty-year-old voted best smile... by me.

~Cristy Trandahl

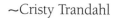

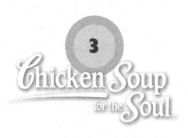

Drop That Spatula

There is no more lovely, friendly and charming relationship,
communion or company than a good marriage.
~Martin Luther

It had become our routine and it wasn't a good one.

Pete came through the door at about five o'clock each evening, right in the middle of my preparations for supper. Relief at the sound of his arrival washed over me. Our two young daughters were filthy from a day in our backyard sandbox and needed a good soak in the tub.

So Pete stopped in the kitchen just long enough to drop off his lunchbox, and I—never breaking my spatula's rhythm—offered him my cheek for a kiss.

Then, up the stairs he trudged, our girls whirling around behind him, chattering happily. And I exhaled into my long moment of peace, with only my spatula to tend to.

Throughout supper, our damp, fresh-smelling daughters continued their chatter as Pete and I managed a word or two to each other in between, and perhaps a wink or a smile.

By bedtime (and by that I mean our bedtime) we were spent. We'd drop off to sleep, then wake the next day and do it all over again.

Our girls were happy and healthy, well-fed and shiny. But our marriage was malnourished and dull.

I'd had enough of our dreary routine. I'd had enough of viewing

Pete as my backup, the other half of our two-person tag team. He was my partner in life and love, not just my partner in chores and child-rearing. It was time to do things differently, and I decided it would start with me.

One fateful day around five o'clock, when I heard the lovely sound of the front door and footsteps, I let the spatula clatter into the pan of whatever-was-sizzling and turned to greet my husband.

Nothing I did was earth-shattering. I grinned, said hello, and opened my arms for a hug. But the earth must have moved for Pete because his face lit up in a wide smile, his eyes sparkling.

I'm not sure if I burned dinner that night, what with my diverted attention and inactive spatula. I don't recall whether the girls got bathed or if they went to bed sandy.

I do know that Pete and I talked and laughed that night. I know that I felt younger, happier, and even prettier. I know (he told me) that Pete felt appreciated, even honored, because for those few moments he was my first priority.

And I know that for every evening since then that I have remembered my resolution to drop that spatula, our marriage has been the better for it, and our daughters have, too. Sand and all.

~Mandy Houk

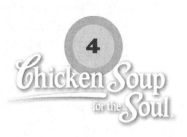

Seize the Day!

I went into the woods because I wanted to live deliberately.
I wanted to live deep and suck out all the marrow of life...
to put to rout all that was not life;
and not, when I came to die, discover that I had not lived.
~Henry David Thoreau

"We are food for worms, lads," declared Professor Keating, the unorthodox English teacher played by Robin Williams in the 1989 film *Dead Poets Society*. "Each and every one of us is one day going to stop breathing, turn cold, and die."

Those words, addressed to his pink-cheeked students, iced the blood in my veins when I watched the movie a few years back. Perhaps it was all in the timing. Only months earlier, I had survived the Big 5-0 and already the New Year was waving a greeting in the near distance. It seemed like the years were passing by while I simply clung to a kite tail. I felt staid, dissatisfied, unfulfilled. In short, I felt my own mortality.

This, perhaps, is why I scooted to the edge of my seat, transfixed and determined not to miss one profound word from the professor's mouth.

"Carpe diem, lads. Seize the day!" he preached to the literature class at the exclusive Welton Academy. "Make your lives extraordinary!"

Later in the movie, the teacher urged the boys to stand on his desk, as a reminder to look at the world in a different way because the universe was broader than their view of it. Everyone, I thought to myself, should have such a bohemian insurrectionary in their lives.

As I inhaled scene after moving scene, the rallying classroom cry, "Carpe diem!" sang in my ears like a mantra. I recognized the words from my four years of high school Latin class, only back then Mrs. Maag had taught the more literal translation of "carpe diem"—"pluck the day."

I liked that image better, I decided. Pluck the day.

Seize the moment.

Or, as Robert Herrick so poetically penned centuries ago, "Gather ye rosebuds while ye may."

Entranced, I sat as the last movie credits rolled down the screen, impulsively reevaluating my life and rethinking my annual goals.

To date, I had lived mostly from the detailed, itemized lists I created annually when the old year faded and the new one offered a fresh start. So dedicated was I to this system that I used to make separate goal lists for each of my four children, another for my husband, and even one for the dog. Why, I was known to make master lists that organized my battalion of lists! Now, however, I knew I needed to make a drastic change.

What would happen, I wondered, if I set aside my lists this next year and took Professor Keating's advice to "suck out all the marrow of life." Could I survive without daily, weekly, and monthly guides to order my hours? Could I still be productive? Reliable? Successful?

And, just that quickly, I resolved to give it a try.

I decided to embrace the unknown. I opted to live life with deliberation. I chose to make my life extraordinary.

But what, exactly, did that look like?

For me, it meant transcending the mundane in order to accept change. I discovered elasticity in me that I never knew existed. I learned to embrace serendipitous opportunities and to discover delight in the moment. Above all, this new outlook left me open to possibility.

Yes, I still dealt with the day-to-day reality of... oh... you know... the kinds of minutiae written on the lists that once consumed me.

But those demands no longer determine my days. Instead, I'm open to chatty phone calls, a spontaneous lunch with a friend, and an evening walk with my husband. I'm freer to entertain, eager to extend an invitation to houseguests, and willing to organize a family reunion. I'm no longer reluctant to travel, to commit to a community project, to volunteer as an election judge.

Now, I focus less on my housework and more on enjoying my home. Instead of worrying about weight, I find pleasure in fresh food and homegrown vegetables. Rather than list all I need to do, I keep a gratitude journal of the new blessings I discover in each waking hour.

So, this New Year, as in the past few, I will make only a single resolution. A resolution I find satisfaction in writing and joy in keeping: Carpe diem!

~Carol McAdoo Rehme

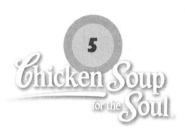

Resolution Evolution

Every day may not be good,
but there's something good in every day.
~Author Unknown

New Year's resolutions—I've made them, broken them, and returned to try again. Whether it was losing weight, eating healthier, or not biting my fingernails, each new resolution began with great determination, only to fade as the days and weeks of the New Year passed.

Last December, I decided to focus on something very different. Through the process, I gained a unique perspective on what matters most in my life and a simple tool that can lead me to greater happiness.

I am the mother of three adult children with special needs, who are still living with us. I have also recently been diagnosed with a neurological disorder that affects my ability to do many of the things that I have enjoyed over the years. It is very easy to become mired in discouragement. I hate to admit it, but I have held several "pity parties" and sadly invited many family members and friends to attend. That is where I found myself last year at resolution-making time. I knew that I needed to do something different.

I started reflecting about the time when my children were young. During those years, my husband and I consciously made a point of remembering what we called "golden moments." The day my son finally learned to tie his shoes, at seventeen, was one of those times. It was definitely a golden moment. During my children's youth, I held tight to the memory of special times, successes, and joys. I tucked them away in my mind to be pulled out later during moments of discouragement, when things were not going well.

So as the New Year began, I resolved to once again consciously look each day for golden moments, for special blessings, for everyday occurrences that led me to a sense of gratitude and wonder. The marvelous thing was they were everywhere!

One day as I was out walking downtown, I became discouraged about my difficulties with walking and my need to use a cane. As I was grumbling to myself, I looked across the street and saw a man in a wheelchair with no legs. This may seem like an overused cliché, but it reinforced for me the fact that perspective plays a pivotal role in my attitude and ability to face adversity.

When I received invitations to friends' children's college graduations, weddings, and baby showers, I felt sad that my children might not experience those same things. But then I reflected that they were all good and caring people who brought great joy to my days. Our life wasn't bad, it was just different.

As time went by, I realized more and more that it was the simple things that were making the biggest difference for me. I found myself pausing to enjoy a beautiful sunset or a mother bird building a nest outside my living room window. I saw a person's kindness as a dear gift.

I guess you could say that I made it my resolution to play the "Glad Game." You know the one, from the movie *Pollyanna*; where even in the most difficult situations, Pollyanna finds something to be glad about. There are probably many people who would scoff and declare this a saccharine-coated way of dealing with life. My answer to them would be, "Why not? Why in this world of trouble and heartache should I not want to consciously choose to seek a better vision, a more grateful heart?"

Am I good at it all the time? Definitely not! I still get discouraged from time to time. I still find the negative creeping back. But the wonderful thing about this type of resolution is that even when I falter or slip a little, I can easily pick it back up again and go forward. All it takes is pausing for a moment to look around me and recognize the simple, pure pleasures and blessings in each day.

~Jeannie Lancaster

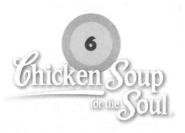

6

System Recovery

Never trust anything that can think for itself
if you can't see where it keeps its brain.
~J.K. Rowling

I hate my computer.

It seems every time I resolve to clear the clutter from my life, my computer crashes. I pull the plug and let the system catnap, a tactic that usually works.

Not today.

I point the arrow to "Start Windows Normally" and cross my fingers. No such luck. I try "Last Known Good Configuration." That's all I want, to get back to where I was before.

That doesn't work either, so I click "Safe Mode." If I can't go back, that's the next best option, right?

Wrong. No matter what I do, I get the advanced options menu.

Desperate, I hit the F10 key. "Do you want to start System Restore?" the dialogue box reads.

With a sigh of relief, I click "yes." A tiny "system restore" box pops up in the bottom left corner. That does not inspire confidence. I want to see "System Restore" splashed across my screen. I want to see the progress bar creeping to the right, like the mercury in a thermometer, apprising me of my status.

Instead, the screen hiccups, spits out line after line of hieroglyphics as if they were watermelon seeds, then blinks back to the menu.

Where is my "Bliss" screensaver? The one with the rolling green meadow and the blue sky?

As I sit here staring at the screen, I realize this is oddly appropriate, since I've gotten stuck in general. The computer is just mirroring my life.

Haven't I been clearing out my life? I gave away most of the books that spilled from my bookcase and stood stacked on the floor. I threw out most of the papers that had multiplied over the years like mold. I donated household clutter to various charities. I even hauled all the stuff stored in the attic out to the curb.

There'd been only one thing left to deal with: the clutter on my computer.

But with the computer, you don't have to worry about being buried alive, like when you open your closet door.

Or do you? I'm beginning to wonder.

I download stuff, intending to get back to it "some day" and actually read it. It takes me whole days at a time to sort through the hundreds of saved articles every few months.

Which, of course, is enough to blow anyone's fuse.

So I guess it only stands to reason that habit would fry my computer's fuse too.

Apparently, it did.

Only one option remains; I know that. When I ventured up to the attic to clear out the broken camera equipment, the mildewed books, the broken projector and fading film, and the Easter baskets left over from my childhood, I found that a friendly family of mice had taken up residence and had left, like the Easter Bunny, "treats."

The internal computer mice are pooping all over my system. My only option is to vacuum. And that means throwing everything out first, just like in the attic.

I hit F10 again to bring up the dialogue box for "System Recovery."

Dialogue, my patootie. There is no dialogue. When your computer throws a temper tantrum, you're out of luck.

Isn't life the same way?

No, I'm in "Wild, Wild West" territory. Shoot first, cry later.

I hold my breath, and hit the "System Recovery" button.

"Are you sure you want to proceed?" the box asks, because System Recovery will erase all your files.

Everything will vanish with the click of a button. But I don't have a choice.

It's showdown time at the OK Corral. I can hear the ominous background music in my head. (I certainly can't hear it on the speakers.) Have I backed up everything critical? I feel like a mother sending her kid off to summer camp for two months, wondering if I forgot to pack underwear.

It's too late now anyway. The bus has left the terminal. But I'm a writer. There are my manuscripts, business records. All my stuff.

What stuff? I can't remember. Just stuff. Like packing peanuts. You don't really know what to do with them, you just save them. Because you might need them someday.

When you could just as easily use crumpled newspaper or plastic bags or popcorn.

I click "Yes."

As the progress bar beeps, I imagine all my stuff—my life—fading into the abyss, sucked away into the vacuum of my computer's space.

And yet, as the bar inches to the right, it reminds me just how far I've come these last couple of years. I've been pruning. I've been deleting bookmarks and files, backing things up, throwing out the clutter. I'd just gotten stuck, and the universe decided to help me along.

The progress bar reads 85% completed. I'd say that's about right.

Up pop the words, "System Recovery complete."

The morning sun is bursting through my window. On impulse, I creep outside to check on a shrub I pruned—brutally—weeks ago. It had gotten so overwhelmingly large; I couldn't squeeze past it anymore. It jutted out across the path and blocked the gate. So, I'd had to cut it back to the main stem. To the core.

Where I'd cut, fresh green buds sprouted.

The same thing happened when I started saying "no" to tasks I really didn't want to do, or to people I really didn't want to be around. I'd pruned the negative energy surrounding my life. I just hadn't hit the delete button on my own negativity.

I think about the computer, filled with articles I'd never gotten around to reading. I'm relieved not to have to wade through those hundreds of files. If they had really been so important, wouldn't I have simply read them online in the first place?

That empty desktop doesn't look so ominous anymore. It is a tabula rasa, waiting for me to write upon it. Like life.

I resolve not to hold onto so much stuff—which is really just negative energy—in the coming year. And if I do, my computer will tell me when enough is enough and it's time for a purge. It will also remind me to embrace quiet time. Those fifteen minutes of "recovery" time forced me to just breathe. I resolve not to wait until my own operating system crashes to "Start System Recovery."

Life is too short to be constantly playing "catch up" with the clutter. You don't need it. And maybe getting back to where you were before isn't the best option to choose. The clutter, be it the past, people, or objects—even emotions—that you've outgrown, stunts the new growth in your life.

The "Bliss" screensaver is back, reminding me to go outdoors and enjoy the sunshine and the freedom of summer.

And to start writing again. Writing something new.

I love my computer again. And my life. I'm moving forward.

~Donna L. Turello

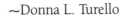

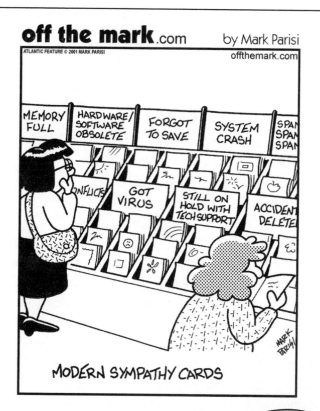

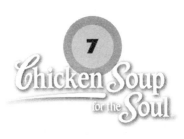

Talks Too Much

We have two ears and one mouth so that
we can listen twice as much as we speak.
~Epictetus

alks too much. Gabby. Chatty. Loquacious. These are all words and expressions that have been used to describe me from the age of four. My mom boasts that I was talking in three and four word sentences before I was ten months old. Some say it's the gift of gab while others simply think I talk too much.

As my thirties came to a close, I found myself reflecting on my life. I'm very happy and have no significant regrets. Even the things that I'm not proud of, I accept as part of my journey to where I am today. When I looked back on those times of difficulty, I saw a clear common denominator; I didn't seem to know when to stop talking. Whether it was hurting someone's feelings, or having carelessly revealed a secret, the incident could have been avoided had I closed my mouth sooner. It was during this life revelation that I resolved to practice the power of quiet.

To take this step, I needed to understand how people could sit comfortably in a group and not talk, and even more amazing, be with just one other person and not talk. Why does my husband feel completely content to sit in a room bustling with conversation and say nothing? He's highly intelligent and has wonderful opinions but he'll sit quietly and just listen. Even when he's asked a pointed question, he'll answer with as few words as he can muster while still communicating effectively. What talent!

Can you imagine being happy just listening? In surveying those I know who talk less than I do (pretty much everyone), the general consensus was one of two answers—they either didn't feel confident enough to speak up and risk being judged on some level, or they just didn't feel the need to participate in the conversation. Of course there were other reasons for not talking, but these were the two most popular answers.

The first one didn't work for me. I'm just fine letting people think what they will about me, and hopefully they'll even speak up and make the conversation that much more interesting. The second one didn't work either. I do feel the need to participate. I feel it physically like an electrical pulse through my body; sometimes it's so strong it causes me to behave badly in the form of interrupting or speaking in an unusually loud voice. I had to look further.

An interesting thing happened on this journey to the power of quiet. During my weekly yoga class (a class I take for the sole purpose of learning to be still), it came to me. Like an answer so crystal clear that the words rang in my head like soft, heavenly bells.

I talked too much so people would know I cared about them. It was my way of taking care of those I love, whether they are family, friends, acquaintances, or customers. I talked so they would know I understood. I resolved before my fortieth birthday, that from that day forward, those around me would know I loved them, and cared what they thought and felt, but I was going to practice the power of quiet.

As my forty-second birthday approaches, I can say that resolving to talk less has been more about focusing on quality rather than quantity. I've found that listening more shows those who I care about that I really do care how they feel. Now when I chime in, it means more to them. Oh sure, I still have my bouts of talking too much, but for the most part this has been one resolution that I can call a success.

~Kathleen Partak

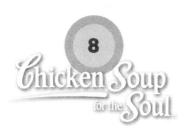

Celebrating a Life

Time is a physician that heals every grief.
~Diphilus

It was almost New Year's Eve 2000, and the nation was getting ready to celebrate the dawn of a new decade. My husband, Don, and I could care less.

In July of 1999, my husband and I lost our beloved twenty-eight-year-old son when he fell asleep at the wheel. He was our accomplished classical guitarist with a master's in music. He was our handsome, blond-haired treasure that could never be replaced. He was a young man with a fabulous sense of humor, a cherished brother to his siblings, and his bright future was cut way too short.

We never were much for New Year's Eve celebrations. Oh, we'd gotten together with friends and raised a glass or two over the years on various New Year's Eves. But the holidays in 1999 and 2000 were some of the toughest days of our entire lives. When you are in early grief, you constantly replay the circumstances surrounding the death of your loved one. It must be nature's way of making it "sink in" and become real for you, so that you learn to live with this in your life. We certainly were changed forever. We felt far from festive as Christmas faded and New Year's Eve rolled around.

My husband and I grieved separately in the early years, trying to spare each other, or minimize the pain each of us was experiencing by not sharing it with each other. It took some time before we could come together and share our tears. I remember going to bed around

8 P.M. so that I would not be reminded of happy people lifting their glasses to toast a new year and a new decade. A new year without my son? A future without him in it? It was too unbearable for me to even comprehend or consider.

Each subsequent New Year's Eve got a little easier, but it was still the policy for me to avoid the group celebrations, the television coverage, and the festivities of New Year's Eves. Who would want to be around me when my mind was fixed on my terrible loss? How could I celebrate living in a world without my son for yet another year?

At some point in time, it happens. You make the switch. For me it was five years after his death. New Year's Eve was approaching. Christmas had been a celebration with family that I truly enjoyed. It was the year that I decorated a small tree with his pictures as a memorial, and it felt right. I hung his stocking that I made him as a child and smiled at the memories it brought me.

I had witnessed an episode of *Dr. Phil* on television where a mother who lost a daughter just could not get over her grief, and it had been TEN years. She was so, so sad and very much STUCK in her grief. I remember Dr. Phil saying to her in so many words, "You had eighteen wonderful years with your daughter, and the only thing that you are dwelling on now is her death. You need to celebrate the wonderful time you had together." The mother looked up at him and said, "I never thought of it that way."

I knew that I was also learning to be thankful for the years I had with my child, the blessing of his twenty-eight years. What if I'd never been blessed with knowing him at all? I realized that I could have lost him as a baby, a toddler, a young child, a teenager... but I was blessed with twenty-eight years!

That year, in 2004, my husband and I resolved to celebrate our New Year's Eve together, remembering and celebrating our Donnie, not mourning him. We looked at photographs and talked about the wonderful times with him.

My husband never made it until midnight, but I did. I stayed awake to welcome 2005, knowing it would be an even better year, because I was learning to go forward with my life. I would always have the sorrow in my life, but it was no longer overwhelming. I could make it my resolution to take forward with me the wonderful memories of my son, the ones that make me smile and subsequently help to soften the pain a little more each year. I raised my glass of wine to God at midnight saying, "Thank you for my wonderful son who blessed my life in so many ways!"

~Beverly Walker

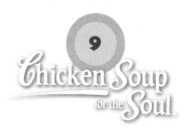

You Are Enough

It's the menace that everyone loves to hate but can't seem to live without.
~Paddy Chayevsky

I started working for CBS when I was nineteen years old and in college, and then I went on to work for NBC. I also assistant-directed two independent features. By age twenty-two, I was employed by one of the largest commercial companies in the world, so the bulk of my work focused on advertising, working on production teams for hundreds of television commercials. I styled and designed ads for *Vogue, Mirabella* and *Elle*, and I worked for Lucasfilm in their commercial division. I was fortunate to experience such an amazing career at such a young age, working all over the country with some of the most creative people in the world. I had it all.

And then one day my life changed.

It was one of those days that you always remember. The sky was blue, and the sky is so rarely blue in Los Angeles. The ocean was sparkling like diamonds and the film set was perfect.

I was filming a diet cola commercial in Malibu.

Then, suddenly, a thought came through me like a lightning bolt. "This is an industry that uses anorexic models to sell diet cola to teenage girls."

And I quit.

A twelve-year career.

Right then.

That night I went home and hit my knees. I did not want to be a part of the problem; I wanted to be a part of the solution. But I had no idea what the solution looked like. So I said a kind of prayer that went something like this—"Right now, with all my gifts and all my insecurities and all my strengths and all my weaknesses... right now—with my skills—what can I do on behalf of the world?"

My grandfather used to say, "Start with what you know, and more will be revealed."

I knew the film, television and advertising industries and almost everything about them.

So I started going into junior high schools. I held up pictures of the models to show what they looked like at five o'clock in the morning, and then held up another picture showing what they looked like after three hours of professional make-up, thirty-five lighting technicians, and professional photographers who can make anyone look beautiful and sexy... not to mention the efforts of post-production, where they airbrush all of the wrinkles, pimples, stretch marks, scars, cold sores and every other imperfection right out of the picture. With digital technology, they can even stretch the models to make them appear taller and thinner.

When the first digital machines came out, I watched my friends learn what they could do. One editor said, "This machine is going to change the world. Anything that we see that we don't like, we can simply change it and make it perfect!" I doubt that he was thinking about the repercussions for our children when he made that statement.

Advertising is powerful. Television is powerful. It is everywhere, and our children are listening to it and watching it. We have to be very careful as adults, because when we talk about our bodies and our diets and all the ways that we are impacted by these ideas, our children are listening. Children as young as five put themselves on "diets." So many children are upset about their bodies.

So I went into the schools and talked to the girls and said, "This is a multi-billion dollar industry that spends millions of dollars a year proving to you that there is something wrong with you so that they can sell you something to fix it. So I am here to tell you that your teeth are white enough... and your breath is fresh enough... and your thighs are thin enough. You are enough. We can no longer afford for the best and brightest among us to live in a state of constant insecurity."

It was interesting because the teachers began asking me to speak at their teachers' conferences and the mothers started asking me to speak at their women's conferences. The next thing I knew, I was speaking around the country on any given day to eleven- and twelve-year-olds during the day and to thousands of women at national conferences at night.

It is thrilling to know that many people are out there now talking about these issues, but back then, in the mid- to late-nineties, no one was really talking about any of this. By the time little girls are ten and eleven years old they have been hit with so many media messages that they are already at the mercy of, and manipulated by, an industry that has gone insane.

While doing my speaking around the country, one day I got the idea "you are on the right track—but you need to start with the babies." I wasn't sure what that meant but I knew it was an important piece of my work. So I took a thirty-three-day road trip in silence to think about it; just me, my car, and my camera. I traveled all through the western United States. At the end of the trip, I ended up spending four days by myself out in the Sedona desert. Sitting out there all alone after thirty-some days in silence, I kept thinking about that idea—"you are on the right track but you need to start with the babies." I am forty-three years old and I spent my first twenty years safe from any idea of a super model floating around in my subconscious.

Today's little girls have never known anything else.

Soon after the trip, I was writing in my journal. It wasn't a particularly interesting entry—something like "yesterday I did blah blah blah," and suddenly I began to write "Cassandra. Cassandra was strolling along. Cassandra was singing a sing-a-long song." And I just kept writing and the entire book came out in one sentence.

Cassandra's Angel is about the stories that we are given from the people in our lives about who they think we are... and then dropping those stories so that we can become who we came here to be.

It is a book about a little girl, Cassandra, who goes through a series of events in which she is collecting all of these "stories"—or negative messages—from the people in her life. It is about how she lets go of the stories that other people have written for her, so that she can make her own story about who she came here to be.

After many rejection letters, I found a small publisher in Washington, and *Cassandra's Angel* won the Best Women's Book of the Year, Colorado Book of the Year, and was a finalist for the International Visionary Award. It experienced record sales with no national marketing—it was all by word of mouth, just like *Chicken Soup for the Soul* in its early days. The book continued to enjoy great success, and has led to a widely acclaimed CD as well. Now *Cassandra's Angel* may even turn into a Broadway musical.

I am often asked who Cassandra is. I didn't know anything about Cassandra when I wrote the book, but learned later that the original Cassandra was the Trojan princess from Greek mythology. Very beautiful, she received a lot of attention from Apollo, who fell madly in love with her and gave her the gift of prophecy. But Cassandra wanted nothing to do with Apollo. So he punished her, altering the gift by taking away her power of persuasion. So there's Cassandra. She knows everything that's going on. She knows the truth. She knows the future, but no one will believe her.

Although Cassandra in my book is vibrantly creative, magical and obviously inspired, the other characters in the story do not honor her gifts. Her journey leads her to a place of solitude where she realizes that her true power comes from within. The final illustration in the book presents a young woman whose powers of persuasion have been fully restored. Cassandra is all young women from all times—strong, vibrant, creative, and sensitive—living in the pursuit of their own truths.

I believe that we all have the truth deep inside us. But each one of us, in our own ways, must make that decision to figure out who it is that we want to be. I have been challenged to my core personally, professionally, and financially many times over since I started this project. I have been on the edge of losing everything more times than I care to admit. But something inside of me would not let me quit. I think we all go through that experience. Fears are going to come up. But it's making the choice to face the fear, to just go through it. I kept telling myself, "I am going to do this, no matter what." There is a kind of profound power available when we commit to something bigger than ourselves.

~Gina Otto

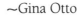

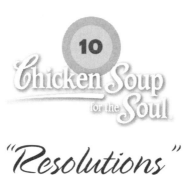

10

Chicken Soup
for the Soul

"Resolutions"

Rest is not idleness, and to lie sometimes on the grass under trees
on a summer's day, listening to the murmur of the water, or watching the
clouds float across the sky, is by no means a waste of time.
~J. Lubbock

This year I will burn a candle and bask in the fragrance of
    spiced apple.
I will take a nap between fresh sheets and not set the alarm.
I will laugh aloud even though there is no one else to hear me.
I will step out in the rain and feel the freshness of spring.

This year I will send a card and tell someone, "I love you."
I will climb hills and fly kites in the March winds.
I will cry at the movies and wish on a star.
I will pray for loved ones, for my country, and the dignity of man.

This year I will run through the tall grass like a giraffe,
    with my head held high.
I will read Shakespeare, Dr. Seuss, and Erma Bombeck
    all in the same day.
I will cradle a soft kitten in my arms and let my soul vibrate
    with its purr.
I will drink amaretto-flavored coffee and eat too much chocolate.

This year I will write love songs, and dance like a child.
I will chase butterflies, rainbows and sunbeams.
I will walk in warm, white sand, and let the breeze
    blow through my hair.
I will walk in the woods and pick wild violets and strawberries.

This year I will ride carousels and eat cotton candy.
I will send flowers to a friend and read to the blind.
I will write poetry and listen to music.
I will take a bubble bath and shop for lingerie.

This year I will rise early enough to see the moon set and
    the sun rise.
I will drive in the country and remember myself as a child.
I will wear pink ballet slippers, perfumed talc, and 14k gold.
I will play in fall leaves and taste the first winter snow on
    my tongue.

This year I will touch more. I will feel the unmatched softness
    of a baby's skin.
I will hold a weathered hand of a friend in the sunset of her life.
I will hug the grieving and feel their pain with them.
And if next year never comes, I've been blessed—
    and touched the hand of God.

~Glorianne Swenson

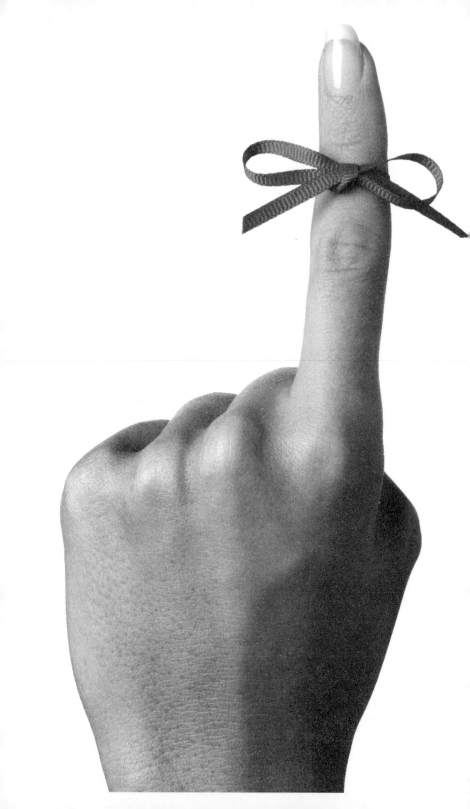

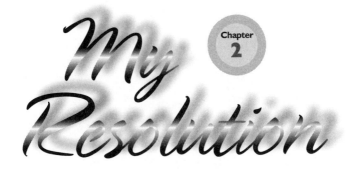

Chapter
2

Anything Is Possible

To dare is to lose one's footing momentarily.
To not dare is to lose oneself.

~Soren Kierkegaard

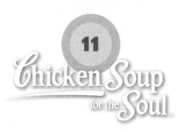

11

It's More Than Just a View

If one dream should fall and break into a thousand pieces,
never be afraid to pick one of those pieces up and begin again.
~Flavia Weedn

As the years have come and gone, like most of us, I've gone head-to-head with a couple of my own personal demons, and in waging those particular wars, I've been known to have made a few resolutions. If the truth be told, I've won some and lost some. Such is life. However, for almost three decades now I've carried with me a bottomless pit of determination to get something back which I truly felt belonged to me.

It all began when I was expecting my first child twenty-seven years ago. My father, deep in the throes of a raging midlife crisis and empty nest syndrome, threw a hissy fit over what were actually a couple of minor annoyances up at the lake, and sold our family cottage. The decision immediately became his greatest regret, and, I believe was one of the only things he died still kicking himself over; besides the fact that my mother didn't speak to him for weeks over it.

My parents had signed for the cottage on a damp and dreary spring morning for not much more than a song. The place was a dilapidated mouse-infested money pit, but it did have a view to die for. I was about to turn sixteen, and in my narrow-minded youth, their decision to buy it was total vindication, as I considered them crazy based on some of the outrageous rules they had devised for me. However, my opinion didn't seem to faze them, and alongside my mom, dad and sister, I toiled away all summer.

By the time my late August birthday arrived, the place was pretty much unrecognizable inside and out, and swallowing my adolescent pride, I asked, much to my parents' delight, if I could hold my birthday bash up there. It was the first of many, as the cottage quickly became the preferred venue for just about every summer family celebration imaginable. Over the years, Mom and Dad bought all the requisite toys, which included a brand new six-seater bow rider and a trail bike. The cottage was the place I first fell in love, and where I learned to drive a boat, a car and a motorcycle, cast my own line, water ski, and play a mean game of croquet and badminton.

Since all of this occurred before global warming or the melanoma epidemic, we also did a fair amount of sunbathing and were all as "brown as berries," as my mom used to say, by the end of summer. Sometimes, craving a little rural excitement, everyone would pile into Dad's station wagon and head to the Country Café in town for lunch. Wandering to our heart's content amongst the little shops along the main street, we'd never fail to make a stop at the bakery. I'm glad no one was testing our blood sugar. By today's standards we should have all been dead long ago!

Evenings were spent toasting marshmallows around the campfire, playing Scrabble, acting out charades or playing family-friendly games of crazy eights, blackjack and every kind of poker imaginable. And during the warmest of evenings, when the moon didn't cast too bright a beam across the cool, dark water, you could almost count on catching the muffled giggles from those who'd ditched their clothes to take a midnight plunge.

We woke early in the morning to Dad popping his head in our bedroom doors advising us to rise and shine if we wanted to eat. Since we hadn't heard of cholesterol counts, we'd show up to the breakfast table and plan the days' activities over platters of bacon and eggs, and toast that was slathered with butter.

Those wonderfully happy times, which I now understand were the epitome of life flying by, were quite simply the best days I have ever known. The second we walked away from that place I truly understood what it meant to have my heart broken.

Unfortunately, I've since learned the hard way it wasn't the only time that would happen, and that at the end of the day there's no prescription for feeling better quick. However, I did make a vow that one way or another; I was going to get it back. I would right my father's wrong and reclaim what was rightfully ours. And so began the grieving process, which, I've decided, is something akin to having the world watch from the sidelines as you take a huge slap in the face, just when you least expect it.

More than a quarter of a century has passed, and my grieving has been somewhat diluted by life's stark realities. However, I kept my promise by diligently monitoring the real estate listings and making a yearly trek up there "just to see," warning my husband that if I ever saw a sign on the property, I'd be willing to post one of the kids on eBay in order to get my hands on it. He responded by giving me the same nervous little smile every time, but to his great relief, it has never once come on the market.

And now, to be honest, I'm tired of waiting. The baby I was carrying all those years ago is about to become a father, which, if you trace the family tree, makes me a grandmother. And yet it's taken all this time for me to grasp the fact that it wasn't about the cottage at all. Or at least not that particular one. What I yearned so badly to recapture and pass on to my own family, was really just a place. A little piece of heaven where the good times we shared, the relationships we strengthened, the lessons we learned and the memories we created would live forever. I hit the Internet a couple of months ago but didn't find what I was looking for until my son sent me the link to a listing. The place, which had a view to die for, was nothing but a dilapidated mouse-infested money pit. We signed the papers within an hour.

Even though it's less than a half-hour drive, I have no plans to travel down the long, dusty road to sneak a peek at the old digs this year. It's been gone almost thirty years now anyway. And I've noticed that with the purchase of our new place, that endless longing and gnawing resolve, which has tugged at my heart all these years, is finally gone. Replaced by an understanding that taking it away from someone else would never have been the answer, I finally learned that it was only in recognizing the cottage's true gifts: the legacy of love it inspired, and the willpower it instilled in me in wanting so desperately to get it all back, could I pay tribute to it. And as I look out at that view and await the birth my first grandchild, I'm almost certain I can see the reflection of Dad's proud smile and the ghost of love's first kiss, in the glistening waters....

~Debbie Gill

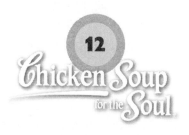

Realizing Impossible Dreams

So many of our dreams at first seem impossible,
then they seem improbable, and then, when we summon the will,
they soon become inevitable.
~Christopher Reeve

Recently, for the first time in five years I made a seemingly simple resolution. I went out back, put my cane down, and started walking. I made it forty-two yards.

That "simple" resolution evolved into something quite powerful and life-changing.

Today I walked five miles.

My medical team had said this would be impossible. My brain could no longer send the signals for walking because those nerves in my spinal cord had been destroyed. Though certainly unintentional, my doctors did take something very important away from me: hope.

A while back, a psychologist pal of mine urged me to try to help myself. I was angry. I said, "They're four of Boston's leading neurologists. They all said I'd never get any better."

"They could have all been wrong."

"They said there's nothing I can do! No rehabilitation. No physical therapy. I'm not putting any effort into trying to walk and then be miserable when I fail."

"Trying is never failure."

I'd get steaming mad at people like her. What did they know? And they came out in droves. I heard various things I should try: a soy-based diet, massage, yoga, acupuncture, positive thinking. All of these well-meaning non-experts believed that traditional medical doctors do not know everything about human potential.

However, there was a common denominator in my friends' advice. And that was the word "Try."

What made me finally resolve to try? The answer is simpler than I'd have ever imagined. That day I tried walking on my own, I said to myself, "Why not?"

When I walk I have a Frankenstein-style gait. I get embarrassed so I explain. I met a gal who said, "Stop excusing yourself. Walk proudly!" She's just one of the many who've taught me that if I open my heart to acceptance, the world is filled with support teams.

I've also resolved to open my obstinate mind and really listen to others, experts or not. This not only fosters my own sometimes-frail belief in my abilities; it fosters faith in miracles.

One morning my husband, Bob, said there was a huge present for me in our driveway. He had researched "bicycles for disabled people." It was a 300-pound cycle for two. The seats were side by side. He could pedal while I sat by him and enjoyed the outdoors again.

Um... did I mention it came assembled with a set of pedals for me too?

Now, hundreds of miles later, after exhausting hours of pedaling along beautiful bike trails, I only wish that we owned stock in Ben-Gay.

Bob needs a tube a day to keep up with me.

Last week he repeated, "There's a huge present in our driveway." He led me outside. "Voilà!" he said. "Oh God," I moaned. Bob dubbed it "The One-Woman Dynamo Power Bike."

"Sweetheart? You know I can't ride a bike on my own."

He laughed sweetly. "I know. And you can't walk either. Then why does the pedometer I bought you have seventy-four miles on it?"

And so, I made a now often repeated silent resolution—a declaration that I am praying others will say to themselves as well. "Yes. I can."

Do you think I love my bike? You bet. Think I love Bob? Of course. Think I love life again after cloistering myself in a self-imposed no-can-do closet? Oy! You have to ask?

How do we find hope when hope seems impossible? Do we simply believe in our hearts, our minds and our very souls that we can beat the odds?

Yes.

Christopher Reeve said, "When we have hope, we discover powers within ourselves we may have never known. Once we choose hope, everything is possible."

His immutable words still ring in my heart and I so hope they will in everyone else's: "And you don't have to be a 'Superman' to do it."

~Saralee Perel

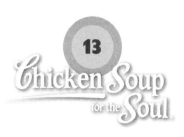

Crazy No More

A New Year's resolution is something that goes in one year and out the other.
~Author Unknown

I was in my usual bind when New Year's Eve came around. It was time to assess the past year and, if there was something I felt needed improvement, to resolve to do better. The familiar candidates came to mind: keep my office neat, stop procrastinating, and get organized. They were familiar because each year I made the same resolutions and each year I broke them. My office was still chaotic, I still waited until the last minute to do things, and organization has become a dirty word.

I remembered hearing somewhere that the definition of crazy is doing the same thing over and over and expecting different results—exactly what I have been doing.

My office was a testament to the craziness. There were piles of papers on my desk and more scattered on the rug. The club chair I placed in there for reading or for the convenience of an occasional guest was dysfunctional. It was more of a magazine rack, laden with so many back issues there was no room to actually sit in it to read. My friends had to sit on the floor. It wasn't pretty.

I assured myself I could—and would—finally clear it up... starting today. I would make my resolutions and stick to them! But first I needed to go to the market before it closed for the holiday. Then on to the cleaners. I promised I would meet my friend later in the day. And somewhere in there I had to make time to work on the writing assignment I had accepted and whose deadline was racing uncomfortably close.

By the time I returned home, I barely had time to put everything away before getting dressed for the evening. My husband and I were going out for dinner with friends. "Let's go," he called. "It's getting late."

I left a cascade of discarded outfits on my bed and rushed out to the car. We came home after midnight. I was too tired to put my clothes away so I pushed them onto the bench at the foot of the bed, tossed the bedspread over them, and crawled under the covers. I was asleep instantly.

In the morning, on the first day of the New Year, I knew I was already in trouble. I took out my journal and wrote the same three resolutions: I will clean my office, I will stop procrastinating, and I will get organized. As I looked around, though, I realized I had already broken all of them. I closed the journal. What was the use? I was overwhelmed by the resolutions. I would never follow them. It was too hard to change old habits. I took my cup of tea upstairs and apologized to my office. "I'm sorry," I told it. "I love you but I just can't keep you neat."

I resented the pattern I had created for myself yet couldn't see my way out of it. In my guilt-ridden wanderings around the room, I brushed against the chair and some of the magazines fell to the floor. Underneath, there was a book I had bought the year before. It was a how-to book on getting organized. I said I would get around to reading it, but not surprisingly, I put it off and eventually forgot about it. Now I suddenly could not wait to read it. It helped me to see that I didn't need to do it all immediately. I could tackle one small thing at a time. I could make a schedule and follow it. I could get organized!

I would start slowly. I could do one project each day instead of trying to do it all at once. I finally knew I could break the pattern. I ran for my journal and crossed out what I had written before. Then I wrote not three, not two, but one resolution. My only resolution this year is to be crazy no more.

~Ferida Wolff

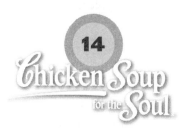

14

Forced to Face the Facts

Resolve, and thou art free.
~Henry Wadsworth Longfellow

"Hey! Why don't you try our pulmonary function test?" The young woman in the American Lung Association booth next to mine tossed her auburn ponytail as she gestured towards her spirometer. The steady flow of customers passing by our displays had dwindled in the late afternoon. "Might as well face the facts and learn if you're up to par."

I cast a wary eye at her equipment. All day I'd been watching people huff into a mouthpiece, and then peer at the results on a printout. Some beamed, but others frowned. I was pretty sure I'd be another frowner. I feared I wouldn't be up to par.

The previous year my father had died. For the last few years of his life he had to make frequent retreats to the bedroom to lie down and breathe with the aid of an oxygen tank. Yet he never quit smoking. Neither had Mom. And, so far, neither had I.

It was mid-December 1984 and the HMO I worked for in downtown Long Beach, California, had staged this wellness fair to provide a service for holiday shoppers and to recruit future enrollees. As a psychiatric social worker, I'd been staffing the mental health display, handing out brochures and fielding questions about stress reduction, anxiety, phobias and, ironically, addictions.

Throughout the day, I'd asked my pony-tailed neighbor to keep an eye on my booth while I escaped to the alley behind the building to grab a quick smoke. She'd smiled sympathetically each time. But now I thought I saw reproach in her eyes as she wagged her hand towards the machine one more time. "Come on," she urged.

My results were about what I had anticipated. I was functioning at about 80 percent of normal capacity for my age and height. Apparently, the aerobic dance class I'd been enrolled in for the past several years had been keeping me fit, but the smoking was definitely taking its toll.

On New Year's Eve I thought about tossing out my pretty pink leather cigarette case with its convenient pocket for my gold lighter. Not yet, I decided. Maybe later. But I vowed to quit smoking.

New Year's Day I scurried around the condo, taking down holiday decorations. Keep busy, I'd told myself. I believed that if I kept my hands occupied I wouldn't need a cigarette. By nine o'clock, I usually had smoked a couple of cigarettes with my morning coffee. This day I had skipped both the coffee and the filter-tips. But by ten o'clock, I gave up. I grabbed my cigarette case and went for a walk. The first drag provided instant relief, and by the time I'd circled the block and stubbed out the butt, I felt better.

As the months dragged by, I would remember my resolution and make new attempts. But cold turkey didn't do it for me. I tried tapering off, the buddy system, relaxation exercises, even affirmations.

I read all the literature that informed me that within five years of quitting, my stroke risk would be reduced to that of a non-smoker. After ten years, my lung cancer risk would be about half that of a smoker's. After fifteen years, my coronary heart disease risk would be equal to a non-smoker. But just as reading diet books hadn't decreased my weight by a single ounce, reviewing these brochures didn't reduce my urge to indulge.

By spring, I'd cut back a little, but not much. I still found myself several times a day huddled under the awning behind the HMO, puffing away while the April showers dampened my hair and sweater.

By early summer, I'd surrendered to despair. Imagery didn't work. No amount of picturing me sprawled on an idyllic hillside or lounging on a tropical beach could counter the intense craving I experienced after more than two hours of not smoking.

Finally, in June, the psychiatrist I worked with took me aside.

"I do hypnosis in my private practice on Saturdays. Come up this next Saturday and let's give it a try. I'll give you a reduced rate."

I trusted this doctor implicitly. I'd tried everything else, so I might as well try this. I nodded.

"If you can imagine yourself as a non-smoker, your subconscious mind will absorb that as reality," he explained. "You'll be able to relax without needing a cigarette."

Saturday morning I gathered up all my ashtrays and put them in a cupboard. I purposely smoked the last cigarette I owned on the drive to his office. The session took less than an hour. The doctor began by putting me in a relaxed state, and ended by giving me some positive post-hypnotic suggestions.

I drove home full of optimism. Upon arrival, I threw away my leather case and lighter.

For the first week, as the nicotine slowly left my body, I felt tingly. I knew it was my nerves reawakening and there was no reason for alarm. After a month or two I no longer found myself glancing about for my cigarette case when the telephone rang. Eventually I learned what to do with my hands when conversing with friends.

Why did it work for me? First, I desperately wanted to quit. I had faced the facts, knew what happened to my father, and seen the printout of my lung test. Second, I believed my doctor, who assured me that hypnosis would put an end to the craving. Third, I reframed my attitude — by quitting smoking I would gain good health, not just give up a decades-long comfort.

Five years later I took another pulmonary function test and learned I had regained all my previously lost lung capacity. Now, well over twenty years later, I marvel at how I remained enslaved for so many years.

Each New Year's Eve, I rejoice in the choice I made back in 1984 to become a non-smoker. And I thank that auburn pony-tailed girl for forcing me to face the facts.

~Terri Elders

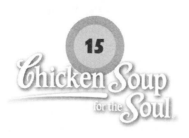

Panic Demons

We acquire the strength we have overcome.
~Ralph Waldo Emerson

Out of the blue, I felt warm sensations creep up from my toes and then start again like waves pulsating through me. My parents' voices seemed to fade into the distance. A terror unlike anything I had ever felt surged through me. I couldn't breathe and my palms began to sweat. My skin prickled and the walls seemed to tilt.

My thoughts ran wild. "My God, what is going on? I am so afraid, but of what? Maybe I'm going crazy. Am I dying? Is this what it feels like? I'm only twelve; I'm too young to die! Something awful must be happening to me, I feel so strange." The waves of panic continued and I wanted to run... run away from this feeling of gut-wrenching fear.

Dad was leaning casually against the kitchen wall, sipping his usual before-dinner cocktail. I think he saw the terror in my eyes as he gently grabbed my arm.

"Sallie, what's wrong with you?"

"I don't know, I feel so weird. I, I, I'm so afraid," I cried out.

"Afraid of what?" he asked.

"I don't know, I don't know," I said as I wrung my hands in agitation and moved anxiously around the kitchen. Time seemed to stand still; everything went into slow motion.

Mom had been busy at the stove preparing dinner.

"Sit down and eat; you'll feel better," Mom said, placing a casserole on the checkered tablecloth. My mother's words brought me back. By now, the panic was subsiding and I began to calm down as I eased into my place at the table. My parents' faces came back into focus and my heart slowed its pounding. I started to feel normal but baffled. What had just happened to me?

I think anyone who suffers from panic attacks can tell you exactly where they were and what they were doing when their first one occurred; they will never forget that defining moment when their life changed forever. It lives in your gut and you remember it clean and clear just like a knife scraping against the bone.

After that night, the panic attacks came every half hour. They always started the same; out of the blue, waves of panic cascading over my body. The rest of that year, I lived in a fog. I became very depressed at my inability to stop them. Certain that I was going crazy, I considered suicide, but always dismissed the idea as not being a solution to my problem. Besides, I wanted desperately to live, just not like that.

My parents were at a loss as to what to do with their daughter who was spinning out of control. I was always anxious and didn't sleep well. I became hyper-vigilant as to what my body was doing, always fearing another attack. My thoughts would run amuck; what if I lost control and did something awful, like jump in front of a car, or scream out loud in church.

By spring of that year, the attacks had gradually stopped. I had no clue what had caused them and so I lived in fear of their return. My teenage life retuned to a somewhat normal state except for my high anxiety.

At nineteen, I married my high school sweetheart and had three children before the age of twenty-six. Along the way, a move from Los Angeles, necessitated by my husband's climb up the corporate ladder, sent the panic attacks back. I didn't feel safe anywhere and I became agoraphobic.

I rode with my husband on his client calls, afraid to stay home alone, afraid to leave the house alone. I waited in the car for him and tried to entertain my three children.

I never ventured more than a three-mile radius from my home. I would take one of my children with me for moral support. That's how low I had sunk. I couldn't let my husband out of my sight, he was my safety net.

My husband stood by me and we both realized I needed help, but from where?

Like a dog with a bone, I gnawed on every option I could find for help. I found a therapist who had me talk and talk. I learned a lot about myself but it didn't stop the attacks. I attended an anxiety group meeting every week for three months run by professionals and yet the panic attacks continued. I hopped from doctor to doctor searching for answers. The drugs they gave me only made me high or had terrible side effects. I found that Valium gave me some peace.

For several years, I managed to live an anxious but pseudo-normal life. I got a college degree and went into the job market. But I was always looking over my shoulder, wondering if the panic demons were following me. I left several jobs when the anxiety of being away from home got to be too much. Soon I was addicted to Valium and had to go through withdrawal. Out of options and out of hope, I hit an all-time low.

Shortly thereafter, as I stood in the local bookstore, feeling despairing and depressed, I picked up a book called *The Anxiety Disease* by Dr. Sheehan. As I began to read, I started to cry and then I eased to the floor in sobs... my condition had a name—panic disorder—a chemical imbalance in the brain. Someone finally knew what I had.

I hunted down a doctor who specialized in treating this disorder and he put me on a specific medication for panic. I learned to help myself with positive self-talk and by pushing the envelope. I tried new things that I once found very scary. Gradually my self-confidence grew and I took on new and bigger challenges. Inside me was hidden a very competent and talented soul just waiting to blossom.

One night not too long ago, my oldest daughter asked me if I felt all those years of my life that I lived in anxiety were wasted. I stopped and thought about it.

I told her no, that I have learned to rely on my own intuition and have come to see that I am just the way God wanted me to be. I wouldn't be as strong a woman as I am today if I hadn't faced the demons in my body and my mind, if I hadn't had the courage to keep trying and never give up. I like myself just the way I am and wouldn't trade my life for anything.

During that time of awakening I worked for the President/CEO's of three Fortune 500 companies and a local councilwoman. I have been president of a woman's organization and spoke to more than 400 people at a local fundraiser. I fly again, something I once found too terrifying to even contemplate.

My friends always surprise me when they call me courageous. I am a woman of confidence and self-esteem but it seems second nature now. It wasn't always that way but there isn't too much that scares me anymore. I guess once you've stared down the panic demons and resolve to conquer them, nothing else quite compares.

~Sallie A. Rodman

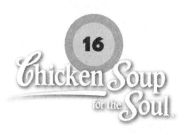

Resolution Revolution

I find television very educational.
Every time someone switches it on I go into another room
and read a good book.
~Groucho Marx

Friends and family constantly ask me how I can possibly find time to do all the things I do. Needing only about five hours of sleep each night helps, but it was a specific resolution that I consciously initiated that really makes everything I do possible.

I'm not sure it was so much a resolution as a revolution. I simply revolted and gave up television, or at least 90 percent of it. I did this near my fiftieth birthday. Perhaps it was a midlife crisis, but I think it was a midlife awakening. I realized that at age fifty either I was well over halfway to being dead, or I was entering a time when more opportunities than ever awaited me, but only if I made changes in my life. I resolved to knock on opportunity's door by making the needed changes rather than to continue pounding on death's status-quo door.

A little math revealed that I had already spent eight years of my life watching television. It added up quickly: an hour or two each morning watching cartoons as a kid; four hours or more in the evening watching news, sitcoms, and movies as an adult, plus weekend baseball and football games. The funny thing is I can only recall a handful of programs from all those years of television watching! I remember seeing Roots—that had an impact. I remember the drama of the space race. I remember the names of a few programs—*Father Knows Best, The Brady Bunch, The Sonny and Cher Show, Star Trek, The Ed Sullivan Show*—but the only things I remember were that I was in love with Cher, and Captain Kirk constantly beamed himself somewhere. The rest remains forever blank.

So is what I've gained by giving up television worth more than what I've missed? I have never seen an episode of *Lost, Sex in the City*, or *Survivor*. Have I missed anything? I think not. I can't remember the last time I watched more than an inning or two of a baseball game or a full quarter of football. Have I missed anything? Nope! Occasionally I watch one of those police drama shows, but I have never experienced any long-term moving experiences or developed even a single noteworthy thought that lingered beyond the closing commercial. And within a day or two I can't even tell you what I last watched, let alone its storyline. I attribute part of my forgetfulness to aging and the associated memory loss, but I'm convinced it has more to do with television's illuminating content—or lack thereof.

What do I do with those extra four or five hours each day? I own a writing business that includes penning books and travel articles, building and maintaining two websites, and traveling for several weeks or months each year. I've been to Costa Rica, Vietnam, Oregon, Washington, Southern California and New England so far this year.

Each spring I plant a huge garden that supplies us with tomatoes, beans, squash, pumpkins, peppers and more. I build furniture in my shop, although the wooden kayak I started five years ago remains hanging from the rafters, half completed. I've remodeled our house, inside and out. I belong to a book club, so I "must" read at least one new book each month, but usually manage two or three.

I take my three-year-old grandson, Jake, for a couple of days each month, and we go out and just have fun. I go on twenty and thirty mile bike rides several times each month. I ride bikes or play games with my stepson Shawn—and help with homework (ugh!) and volunteer at his school. During the past two years I've taken guitar lessons, piano lessons and voice lessons and continue to enjoy all three — although my family is less entertained by my practicing than I am.

While I have no idea what I last watched on television, I do remember what my grandson Jake and I did together last week; I remember the songs I have written and learned to play on my piano and guitar. I remember our travels in Vietnam and Costa Rica and the three weeks I spent driving 5,000 miles throughout Oregon and Washington this summer researching a new book. I remember the book I just finished reading for my book club.

I haven't made a New Year's resolution since my television revolution ten years ago. Having significantly reduced television in my daily routine, I figure I have added at least six years to my life to do the things that I really want to do, things that I will fondly remember well beyond the last commercial — but wait, there are no commercials in my life. Can't beat that!

~Ken McKowen

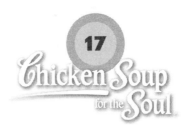

17

The Write Way: Write Away!

The worst enemy to creativity is self-doubt.
~Sylvia Plath

A Step Back

Sweat was coursing down my forehead, falling in tiny drops, smearing the ink of my notebook pages. My heart was a sprinter, with a finish line that seemed to get farther and farther away. Here I was, in the second year of my Bachelor of Education degree, in writing class—and today, it was my turn.

The professor picked up my portfolio and loudly announced, "Today, we'll be critiquing the work of... Charles Baker." Those who knew me turned to look at me and smile. Others soon saw the direction of the stares, and within a few seconds, eyes singled me out. I blushed and slid down a few inches in my seat.

The teacher selected a piece at random. He put the overhead sheet on the projector for all to see. When I looked up to see which piece he had chosen, I breathed a sigh of relief—he had chosen my best poem.

Then my dream became a daymare.

"The first problem with this is... The next thing wrong with it... What the writer hasn't thought about at all is... And can you believe... I'm not sure the writing world is ready for you yet, Mr. Baker."

Nowhere to hide. The eyes that glanced back had different looks now, ones filled with pity, sympathy, curiosity, and in some cases, fear — knowing their turns to trip up would come soon as well.

I made two vows in that moment: never to pick up a pen again, and never to treat my future students the way I'd just been treated. I kept those vows for nearly ten years....

A Step Up

When I decided to earn a second diploma and was registering for classes, I was thrilled to see that I got into all of my main courses, but the electives I wanted all seemed to be filled. I was running out of choices, and then one blinked back at me like a neon sign — a writing course.

I took a deep breath and punched the class code into Telereg. It might be full too, I silently hoped... but then I got the confirmation. I was in. What had I just done?

A Step Forward

To say that this writing class was "a bit different" would be like saying Shakespeare could "string together a few words." We had speed contests with our teacher. He'd write with us, and then those volunteered would read out the drivel they'd written and laugh with the rest of the class.

"It's okay to write garbage," he told us. "I write garbage all the time — sometimes pages and pages of it, and sometimes entire journals of it. But then along comes that one idea!"

He read one of his more polished works, a piece about growing up in a small town. It was powerful poetry that moved us all. Then he showed us where it had come from. He read three pages of a journal of truly horrible writing — words my previous teacher would have reveled in tearing apart. From hundreds of words, he pulled out one six-word phrase that he liked — the words that had led to his masterpiece.

I was encouraged. I found my energy. I wrote more for him in that class than I had in all my previous years of schooling. I wanted to write; I wanted to find words that could move. I made two new resolutions: to never put down my pen again, and to publish a piece of writing.

No Turning Back

The rejections flowed back to me in a constant stream, but my professor just called them "proof that you're writing." He showed me a binder with what must have contained a hundred or more rejection letters of his own. "When you have this many, then we'll talk again."

I didn't have to wait that long. The pressure was off, and I was free to write about what mattered to me. I decided to try a short humor piece about the worst date I'd ever had. When the story was published in a local newspaper with a circulation of over 200,000 readers, and they paid me for it on top of all that, something changed. I caught my second wind for writing.

Since then, I've published hundreds of magazine articles, a collection of poetry, and other fiction and nonfiction books — and, better yet, I've become a writing teacher.

This year, I've had the best surprises of all. One of my grade eleven students won a national writing contest, and one of my grade twelve students learned how to plan a novel in October, wrote 50,000 words of it in November, finished it over December holidays, and sold it to a publisher a few months later. It was published this past summer and is one of more than eighty published works that my twenty-six writing students wrote in a single term.

I've become the writing teacher I always wanted to be, and best of all, I've inspired others to want to write too. We've crossed that finish line together now, hundreds of my students and I... and we can't wait for the next race. There's no turning back now.

~Charles Baker

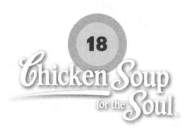

18

Every Little Bit Helps

There is hope if people will begin to awaken that spiritual part of themselves,
that heartfelt knowledge that we are caretakers of this planet.
~Brooke Medicine Eagle

The holiday season was coming to a close and the new year was approaching quickly. I was so pleased with the resolution my family and I had made at the beginning of this year and especially proud that we were actually able to keep it. For the past year we had made an effort to go green and, looking back, I knew we were pretty successful.

Last year we began recycling all of our glass, paper, plastic, and aluminum cans. We changed all light bulbs throughout our home to those energy saving bulbs; we stopped purchasing bottled water and began using SIG bottles. In addition, we made it a point to use reusable bags when grocery shopping; even taking my reusable bags to the mall.

One of the best things we did was to subscribe to a service called Green Dimes. For a small fee, Green Dimes will stop all that annoying junk mail that arrives in the mailbox and use part of the fee they charge to plant trees in the community. Just think of all of the trees we helped save and all of the trees we helped to plant!

Although I was proud of all the changes we had already made, I felt that we could take it a step further for the new year and do more. I was especially interested in teaching my kids, who could always use a good lesson in giving back, to become more involved in learning how important it is to take care of the environment. I began thinking about ways I could further the connection. It took awhile for it to come to me but when it did I was inspired and excited about it.

I figured that, in our own way, we were already giving back to Mother Earth. But wouldn't it be great if we could give more to organizations that support causes which help the less fortunate around the world? What I decided to do was take the money we earned from recycling our aluminum cans, glass, and plastic and give it to charity. We would give to a different charity each time we collected the cash when we turned in our recyclables.

My seven-year-old son, Brayden, would even be able to join in, as he was responsible for sorting the items and taking them to the recycling center with me. I wanted him to become even more involved, and so I decided that he would help me decide which charity to support. He could help to do the research about the various charities on the Internet. Because we cashed in our recyclable items every month or so, we wouldn't have a large lump sum; but I loved the idea of teaching my son that it doesn't matter how much you give; what matters is that you give. The smallest donation can make a difference.

As this year comes to a close we are all proud of the steps we have taken to make a difference. And next year, although the dollar amount won't be huge, we will be doing our part to help the environment and make this world a better place. All of the changes we make don't have to be huge, but if everyone became involved, just think of the difference we could make.

~Laura Dean

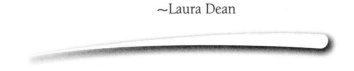

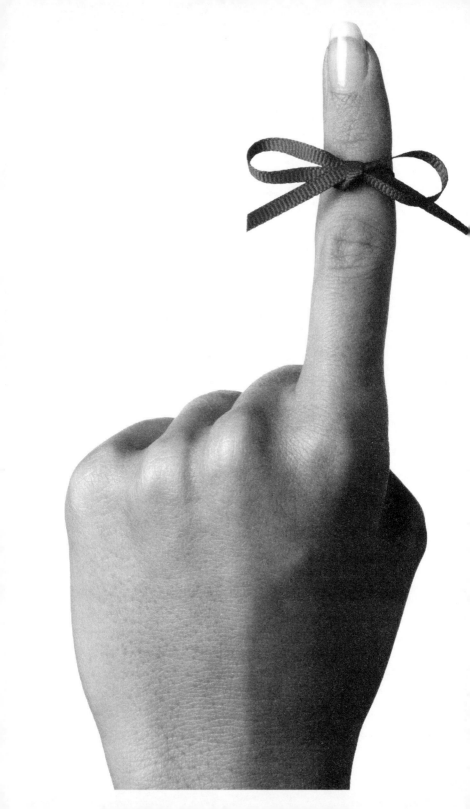

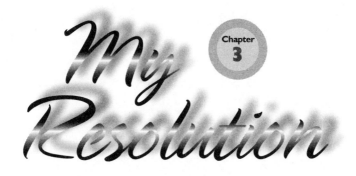

Chapter
3

A Guiding Hand

How far you go in life depends on your being tender with the young, compassionate with the aged, sympathetic with the striving and tolerant of the weak and strong.
Because someday in your life you will have been all of these.

~George Washington Carver

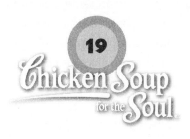

Laundry Prayers

If you want children to keep their feet on the ground,
put some responsibility on their shoulders.
~Abigail Van Buren

have never prayed for laundry before. That is until this morning. It all stems from my closet addiction to doing too much for my kids. Don't look at me all pious. You know you've done it yourself. Of all the things I do for my kids, the hardest by far are the things I force myself not to do. Cooking and cleaning and schlepping the laundry are easy. Not cleaning my kids' rooms but insisting they do it themselves is hard. Running around like a chicken with my head cut off to make sure they get to school on time is easy. Allowing them to be late and suffer the consequences is hard.

I know I'm not the only mom who's stood in my child's toxic dump of a room and thought that I could pick it up myself. It'd take me about ten minutes, all the while knowing that the right thing to do is go find that child, drag his little backside in there and insist he clean it up himself, listen to him whine about how it's not fair, how his sisters never do anything, how he could run away and nobody would care, then have to drag him back three times until the job is done correctly. That's hard!

Actually, I've gone both ways. There have been days when I was just too tired to fight the battle and did the work myself to have it over and done with and days when tough love prevailed, I was willing to be the bad guy, and insisted my child do his own work for his own good. There've been days when someone called to say, "Quick! Bring me my homework (flute, lunch, P.E. clothes) I forgot at home." I clenched my teeth and declared they'd have to do without; and then there were days when I high-tailed it up to school—Mom the enabler.

This year, our oldest child, Haley, started high school—countdown to independence. Loving her enough not to do too much for her seems more immediate now and the goal I am striving towards. In four short years, she'll be at college somewhere trying to figure out how those clean clothes magically appeared in her dresser. Where are the elves that used to vacuum her room? And exactly how did her shoes find their way from the middle of the den floor to her closet while she slept? It's time to rein myself in and start letting Haley take care of Haley no matter how much I still love doing it for her.

That's why yesterday, after I'd issued my "last call for laundry" three times and then discovered a sea of dirty clothes on Haley's bedroom floor, I calmly let her know, "I'm finished washing for today, Sweetie. If you want clean clothes, you'll have to wash them yourself." I didn't get much of a reaction from her, mainly because she's known me long enough to assume it was only lip service. But I really meant it this time. At least, I hoped I did.

I doubt if Haley gave those clothes a second thought as she waded through them on her way to bed last night, but I thought about them for hours. They were the last thing on my mind when I fell to sleep, and the first thing on my mind when I woke up this morning.

Two hours until the bus comes. I still have time to wash and dry a couple loads before then. So I start laundry praying. "Lord, please help me not to wash Haley's clothes. In a few minutes when she wakes up and pitches a hissy fit because she has nothing to wear to school, help me remember why I'm doing this. Thank you for loving me enough to not bail me out of all my messes. I know it must be hard for You to sometimes watch me standing knee deep in 'another fine mess' I've made. Do You ever want to reach down and fix it for me, just this once? I know You want me to be happy. Thank you for loving me enough to let me be miserable, when it's for my own good. Help me to understand that kind of love and please, please, Lord, help me not to jump up, run in there, and wash Haley's clothes for her. Amen."

~Mimi Greenwood Knight

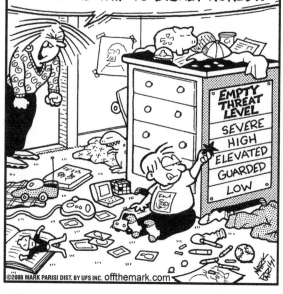

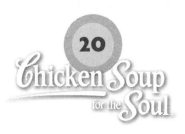

20

A Resolution Gone Awry

It is impossible to keep a straight face in the presence of one or more kittens.
~Cynthia E. Varnado

One steamy July afternoon in central Arkansas, I was working on an important project in my home office with a dear friend and colleague. My trusty printer was churning out a time-sensitive report when it simply stopped. After fifteen minutes of trying to coax, cajole and tickle the device back into operation, we conceded defeat and left to get some lunch and buy a new printer. Upon our return, my heart froze to see the cul-de-sac teeming with fire trucks, a web of hoses, and heavily-suited emergency personnel sprinting toward my house.

Despite having spent much of my life crafting prose, I still stumble for adequate words to describe the sick, sinking feeling of seeing your home, business, and belongings going up in flames along with photographs and memories collected over a lifetime. But the panic that filled my stunned heart in that awful moment was for the nine cats that shared my home after being rescued from situations of abuse and abandonment.

Responding to an early security-system alert, the amazing fire-fighters arrived in record time, but the chemical-laden smoke had already taken its toll. I examined, cuddled, and kissed each cat goodbye, immensely grateful that they had passed gently, without injuries or burns. A dog-lover EMT and the fire chief, who professed a cat-loving wife, assured me they had only taken a couple of breaths before passing. My fur babies had all been found in places they frequented during the day—snuggled on my bed, cupped in a cat tree, nestled on a window sill, and one was even discovered in his favorite hidey-hole behind a 1911 H.P. Nelson upright piano.

Only animal lovers really understand the incredible impact that the loss of one beloved four-legged family member can have on your heart, mind and soul. The loss of so many dearly loved critters sent me reeling.

After staying with another great friend for a couple of weeks, I was relocated to a furnished apartment; rebuilding the house would take months. Overwhelmed by indescribable grief, I made the absolute resolution not to even consider taking in more animals (which friends immediately began to offer) until after returning home, if then. I simply did not have the wherewithal to deal with myself, much less anyone or anything else! The jagged holes in my heart needed time to heal.

The weeks that followed were incredibly rough. It was a time when a maze of critical decisions loomed—securing a contractor, negotiating city permits, maneuvering through cumbersome red tape and over complicated insurance hurdles, replacing everything from toothbrushes to computers, reconstructing tax records, and trying to salvage my business. It was also a time for reassessing my workaholic lifestyle.

One evening, about a month after moving in, I was ensconced in writing a mystery novel (another resolution) when a falsetto "meow" sounded from outside the apartment door. Was it my mind playing tricks again? More than once I had heard, seen or felt the brush of one of my departed furry roommates. The meow grew louder and more insistent. Curious, I opened the door.

Sitting on the doorstep was a kitten with an exotic black coat and alert amber eyes. A neighbor walking by scooped him up and began petting him. When I remarked how cute her kitten was, she explained that he had been born under a bridge in the apartment complex and scrounged around for food. This kitty-loving neighbor was quick to offer an extra litter box if I was interested in giving him a home. My immediate reaction was a facetious "that's all I need!" After all, my resolution had been well reasoned and remained firm.

As if they had conspired like some pre-coordinated team of flim-flam artists, she put the adorable kitten down. Without hesitation or respect for privacy, the little guy sauntered past me into the apartment with a master-of-the-manor air. He took a brief self-guided tour, sniffed here and there, and then curled up on the couch; apparently the residence had passed his inspection. For the first time in what seemed like forever, I genuinely laughed. Not giving me a chance to object, my conspiratorial neighbor appeared with a litter box and enough food for a few days. Wondering when someone had embla-zoned a big "SUCKER" on my forehead, I thanked her and closed the door, resolved to just let him stay until a real home could be found. It is mind-boggling how easily one can become steeped in sheer denial!

That night, as I slid between the sheets of the still unfamiliar bed in the still unfamiliar apartment, the feisty little furball plopped onto the bed, yawned dramatically, and nestled by my side. Those who have never shared a snooze with a critter or two may not relate, but that was the first night since the fire that I actually slept. Stubbornly determined not to open myself to more animals—to more pain—I had refused to admit how desperately I missed having a warm fuzzy cuddled close.

Needless to say, the cat community knew the precise prescrip-tion for healing far better than I. Over the next few days, the kit-ten's hilarious, playful antics drew laughter and affection, in spite of the awful grief tugging at my heart and constant self-reminders he was only visiting for a few days. The name Starlight (Star for short) seemed perfect because that night he brought some light back into my life.

Star grew into a sinewy, sleek black panther-like cat with intel-ligent eyes the color of sun-kissed bronze. Actually, cat is a misclas-sification for Starlight; he's really more like a dog. He craves attention, knows no boundaries, greets workmen at the door, sports a relent-less shoe fetish, harasses his fellow felines, and even plays fetch if in the mood. He adores wrestling rubber bands, races up and down the stairs, darts outside anytime the door opens, suddenly appears everywhere I don't want him to be, holds onto the broom while I'm trying to sweep, rolls in catnip or whatever else happens to be on the floor, and upends every open vessel containing liquid. In hindsight, a better name might have been "Star, Stop It!"

In the five years since the fire, we have been through a lot, Starlight and I. We returned to the house, managed to keep the business alive, replaced belongings as best we could, brought the mystery novel to the final edits before it's submitted in hopes of publication, and made a lot more resolutions. Star helped me through a massive, albeit untraditional, healing of spirit. The memories of the kitties that passed in the fire now spark only warmth in my heart and winsome smiles. Every single day, I appreciate the serendipitous nature of the Universe that sent me hope in the form of a little black furball.

So take a little advice from my furry friend: no matter how bleak things may become or how fixed your resolve may be, open the door whenever opportunity knocks. It just might be a star to light your way.

~Nancy Sullivan

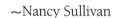

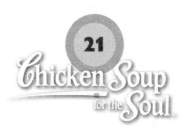

21

You'd Never Know

Today, give a stranger one of your smiles.
It might be the only sunshine he sees all day.
~H. Jackson Brown, Jr.

I was back at the radiation lab. It was time for my yearly check-up.

Sitting there in the office, I remembered the cancer treatments, and the first time I had walked into the lab. My legs felt like tissue paper. I had looked down the long hallway and could only imagine the torture due me. This was a world I never expected to enter. I felt nothing but fear for what lay ahead.

What lay ahead was not as bad as I thought. In fact, the experience brought the unexpected reward of self-discovery. But I didn't know it then. All I knew was that I had been operated on for cancer and now was to undergo five weeks of radiation. My mood showed in my appearance. No make-up. No interest in the clothes I had put on that morning. No smile on my face.

A stunning woman had walked into the building as I waited for my treatment. Stockings, suit, hat, make-up; impeccable.

"I'm here for my check-up," she said, smiling.

I turned to my husband. "You'd never know," I whispered. She had cancer and she looked beautiful. She had undergone radiation and she was walking, talking, smiling, and joking with the receptionist. She was a survivor. I was grateful to see her face and to hear her cheerful voice. It made my legs stronger when it was my turn to go inside for my treatment. I resolved right then and there to someday have her attitude. "I'm going to do for someone else what she has done for me," I vowed to myself.

Now it was one year later. I was back for a check-up.

"How are you doing?" the receptionist asked.

I had dressed in my special clothes. I had washed my hair and carefully applied my make-up. I had been determined to look my best. My new "after cancer" attitude was obvious.

"You look great," she said.

A man was sitting to my right. His face was pale and lifeless. He owned the tissue-paper legs. I knew it was his first time. You could tell. He looked at me for a long time and I knew what he was thinking. I sent a smile his way. His face brightened and he returned it.

I had done my part.

~Harriet May Savitz

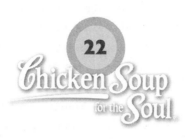

The Doorman

Hugs are the universal medicine and a handshake from the heart.
~Author Unknown

On a road trip to California's breathtaking North Coast region, my hubby Ken and I, my teenage daughter Lahre, and my nine-year-old son Shawn, stopped to have lunch and stretch our legs a bit.

As we walked toward the restaurant's entrance, a gruff looking man jumped up from a nearby bench and opened the door for us. "Good afternoon and welcome to Denny's," he said in a very jovial voice. In his hand he held a ceramic mug full of steaming coffee—which was inviting on such a cold day—but from the looks of the rest of him, it appeared that he hadn't had a good meal or a shower in a long time.

With a scraggly beard and dirty hair that went well past his shoulders, it was obvious he was homeless. An old bike loaded down with a sleeping bag and the rest of his earthly belongings rested against the bench, and his clothing told of hard times, from a weather-beaten jacket right down to his old boots with mismatched laces. But regardless of his appearance, he greeted us as if we were his best friends, adding as we entered, "Today's soup and sandwich special's a great deal."

Once inside, my teenager whispered to me, "Mom, he smells." And Shawn asked questions about him, not quite understanding the concept of a homeless person. After we ordered our lunch, Ken and I explained the best we could, telling the kids to look beyond the dirt and grime to the person underneath and within. As we explained, the four of us watched other customers approach the restaurant; they appeared unsure of the homeless man and many snubbed him or ignored him.

Seeing this rudeness truly frustrated me. The day I became a mother, I had resolved to set a good example for my children. Granted, some days, when things just didn't go right, being a good example was tough.

When our meal arrived, I realized that I had left the car-sick pills in the glove compartment. With the windiest part of our trip just ahead of us, the kids needed to take their medicine. I excused myself from the meal and went to the truck.

As I neared the front door, the "doorman" was opening it for an older couple and welcoming them to the restaurant. They rushed past him and didn't even acknowledge his presence. I let the couple come through first and then said a loud and gracious "thank you" to the doorman as I exited. He teased me by asking if I was running away from my family, and I told him I needed to get something from the truck. When I returned, I showed him the car-sick pills and he laughed, saying he had ridden his bike that direction once and understood the need for the pills.

We talked a bit longer. He told me that the restaurant's manager wouldn't let him inside unless he purchased food. All he could afford was coffee (which, he said, didn't count as "food" according to the manager), so he had to stay outside. But he learned that if he stayed close enough to the front door, the wait staff would sneak out and refill his mug.

I went back inside and told his story to my family. I then asked our waitress, who was bringing the kids their dessert, to add one soup and sandwich special to our bill. Both the kids looked at me funny — as we had already eaten — but Ken knew exactly what I was doing. The waitress was confused, too, but when I explained the order was for the doorman, and that he was to eat his meal inside with the rest of the customers, she smiled and thanked me.

Both children asked why I would order a meal for the "smelly guy." Again, I shared that everyone has goodness inside of them regardless of what they look like or even smell like, and by expressing one simple act of kindness to a fellow traveler in life, the world could possibly become a better place.

By this time, we had to get back on the road to stay on schedule. But before we left, a visit to the "happy room" was necessary to relieve our bladders. As we rounded the corner of the very full restaurant, the doorman was sitting at a table enjoying his meal. When he saw me, he jumped up and thanked me profusely for the hot meal. He then extended his hand for a handshake, which I gratefully accepted. It was then I realized he had tears in his eyes—tears of gratitude.

What happened next drew gasps of astonishment from the restaurant customers, staff and even my own children: I gave the doorman a hug. Just as surprised as the rest of the crowd, the doorman held me tight for just a few moments. Pulling away, his tears were now streaming down his face, and others were beginning to cry, too.

While we can't choose many things in life, we can choose when to show gratitude, and I was doing just that. I was saying thanks to a man who had simply held open a door for me, and also saying thank you for that opportunity to teach my children by example. Hopefully, when someone opens a door for Lahre and Shawn during their journeys through life, they will remember to say thank you. And hopefully they'll have a great soup and sandwich special on the menu, too.

~Dahlynn McKowen

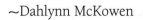

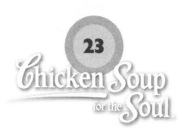

Gifts Year-Round

Yes, God will give you much so that you can give away much,
And when we take your gifts to those who need them they will break out into
thanksgiving and praise to God for your help.
~2 Corinthians 9:11

Last year, I didn't have the heart to disassemble our artificial tree covered in miniature white lights. Each time we passed the living room, we'd pause to gaze at the illuminated corner, a poignant reminder that Christmas is all about giving.

Then, something significant happened each time we looked at that tree.

It reminded us to give a gift to someone each and every day of the year.

One afternoon, our six-year-old neighbor, Hayden, popped in for a visit. As he entered the living room, his eyes instantly spotted the lit tree.

"Wow! A Christmas tree! Why do you have a Christmas tree up in the middle of summer? Christmas has been over for a long time now!"

"We like to celebrate Christmas all year long!" I smiled. "Just this morning, there were a bunch of presents under that tree."

"Where are they now?" he asked, curiously. "Oh, that's one of the rules about celebrating Christmas all year long! Since it's a giving tree, the presents aren't allowed to stay here for more than a day. It's our job to see that they are given as soon as we hear of a need! That's what Jesus would want, right?"

Hayden tilted his head to one side and gazed up at me in wonder. "What kind of presents are they?"

"Well, let me think; one day, we packed up some clothes we no longer needed, and sent them to hurricane victims, and to people in other parts of the world, who aren't as lucky as we are. Of course, we always place them under the tree the night before and pray for the people who will be receiving our special surprises. Another time, I crocheted some soft baby blankets. We wrapped them up in pretty paper, and gave them to a place downtown that could use them. Then there was the day we wrapped up all of our old *Guideposts* and *Angels on Earth* magazines, and took them to an assisted living facility. There are just all kinds of people out there who could use a pleasant surprise, not only at Christmas time, but all year-round!"

The room suddenly grew so quiet; I had to look in Hayden's direction to make sure he was really still sitting next to me.

Suddenly Hayden's face glowed as brightly as the Christmas lights on the tree. "If I go home and color a bunch of pictures, would you wrap them up and give them away as presents?"

I reached out and gathered Hayden softly in my arms. "I think that's a sensational idea! I know that will make Jesus happy too!"

"And maybe we can tell others to keep their trees up all year-round, so they remember that every day is Christmas, right?"

"I'll be sure and let them know." I whispered around the sudden lump in my throat. "Merry Christmas, Hayden!"

"Father, may we keep the spirit of Christmas in our hearts year-round. Help us to teach our children that the reason we give, is because you asked us to. Thank you for sending us the greatest gift the world has ever known, Your Son. Amen."

~Mary Smith

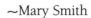

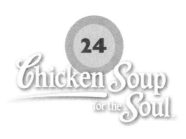

24

You Can Do This

It's not who you are that holds you back,
it's who you think you're not.
~Author Unknown

While many young women growing up in the 1960s chose to break free from traditional career expectations, I accepted the age-old restrictions with little protest. In my "neck of the woods," few young women left the area for job advancement. We chose fields that were available and acceptable in our community, and our educations and training reflected these choices. Limited expectations coupled with a heaping helping of fear and insecurity were more than enough to keep me from being a dream seeker.

Then in the early 1980s, I gave birth to a little girl. She was bright, inquisitive and energetic, and she approached the world with arms open wide. As I watched her grow, I resolved that she would not be handicapped by the mindset that had restricted me. I wanted her to experience her potential, and in the years that followed, often encouraged her personal growth with the words, "Honey, you can do this!"

However, an interesting problem arose during her high school years. Although I had raised my daughter to be fearless and secure, I was quite fearful and insecure when it came to the unfamiliar. Her four years at a large state university helped me to acclimatize to her expanding world, but upon her graduation, she packed and moved to Boston, which was fifteen hours away from our southern home. And while I knew that she could be anything she wanted to be, I just wasn't sure that I wanted her to be so darned convinced that I was right about that. I had always been a "be in before dark, locked door" kind of country girl. I knew nothing about living in cities, I didn't like traveling alone, and I definitely didn't like the thought of my daughter doing either. But her dream was to be a doctor, and my dream was for her to live her dream, so I didn't protest... much.

Her dad and I helped her with the move; then I returned home to worry. In the months that followed, I tried to keep from thinking about her taking public transit late at night. I constantly (and sometimes unsuccessfully) fought the urge to ask, "Did you lock your doors?" And I tried to keep from hyperventilating into the phone when she related any of a number of somewhat scary incidents. But whenever she called to express doubt about her ability to meet the academic challenges, I always responded, "You can do this," because I knew that she could.

Then came the day of her simple and frightening request. "Come visit me without Dad." For weeks she begged, and I offered transparent excuses, but she would not give up. Finally, I relented, packed my bags and flew to my daughter's new home. This was an act of great love on my part because I not only was afraid of cities, I also was afraid of flying.

But my daughter, knowing my fears (and poor sense of direction), met me at the airport and protectively sheltered me throughout the visit — in a challenging sort of way. We explored the city; I had always avoided cities. We went out at night; I had never been a go-out-at-night person. We took public transportation; my prior knowledge of mass transit was the Kingston Trio's 1960s song "M.T.A." in which "Charlie" never returned from his ride beneath the streets of Boston. In the song, Charlie couldn't pay the "one more nickel" increase in fare; but I felt certain that if Charlie, a native urbanite, couldn't escape the subway, how much worse the plight might be for little ole rural me.

Knowing my fears, my daughter inconspicuously clutched my

arm in the subway terminals, and she explained the confusing city traffic to this novice pedestrian. She hovered protectively, and she never left my side until my last day when she had to return to class. But even then she handwrote the exact words I was to say when I phoned for a taxi. How did I get to be fifty years old without ever having requested a taxi? I suppressed the fleeting thought that maybe I needed to get out more.

Not content with my one solo visit, several months later, she was begging me to return. She was the one that I had resolved to set free; why did she keep trying to pull me along, too? "Please, Mom. You can do it," she begged. I sighed loudly. "Don't you want to spend time with me?" Now was that really a fair question for her to ask? Of course I wanted to be with her... but not in a city. Overnight I pondered my dilemma, then booked another flight.

We spent time together exploring sights and sounds that I hadn't experienced before, and I must admit that I felt more comfortable during this visit. In fact, amazingly, I had a great deal of fun. Then the day came that she raised an eyebrow, and then raised the bar.

"I have class this morning," she said, "so you need to take the subway this afternoon and meet me downtown at a coffee shop near the school." My eyes grew wide. She was too young to know about the Kingston Trio's tale of Charlie's never-ending nightmare on the M.T.A. But that was no excuse. She knew that I didn't like cities (well, maybe Boston had grown on me a little). But had she forgotten that I have absolutely no sense of direction and that fear is my sixth sense? What if I never returned... just like Charlie in the song? Then she'd be sorry for misplacing her miserable mother beneath the streets of Boston.

"Mom, you can do this," she said encouragingly, in much the same tone I had used when she was a little girl. "I'll draw you a map," she added, sounding cheerful yet resolute. Placing a detailed drawing in my hand, she hugged me goodbye and hurried off to class.

Of course, I wanted to spend the afternoon with her, but I was still fearful of urban life. Alone in her apartment, I listened to the intimidating sounds of the city and gradually resolved that I would accept her challenge. At midday, I drew a deep breath, locked the door to her apartment and caught the subway... all by myself.

Clutching her map, I navigated to our meeting place then sat down at an outside table to wait. She was running late, and when she finally appeared, there was urgency in her stride as she moved toward me, so I stood and called out, "I did it!"

Her worried facial expression dissolved into obvious relief (or maybe it was pride). It was then that I realized that she had a resolution of her own making. "I knew that you could," she said.

~Joan McClure Beck

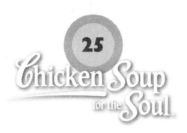

25

The List

He is a wise man who does not grieve for the things which he has not,
but rejoices for those which he has.
~Epictetus

In the days surrounding my grandmother's death, my family gathered to remember her and comfort ourselves by sharing our stories of what she meant to us. One of my favorite stories was told to me by my Aunt Chris.

My grandmother had stopped in to visit Aunt Chris (her daughter), as she was unpacking her belongings in her new house. My aunt had an enormous list of "things to do" posted on her refrigerator; an endless reminder of all the work still to be done for the move. As my grandmother read over the list, she said "Chris, you really should put up another list."

My aunt was exasperated, standing in her new kitchen, amid a mountain of boxes and crumpled newspapers. Every cupboard door and drawer was open. "Another list! Why?" Chris was worried and overwhelmed. "Did I forget something?"

"You should always have a list of all the things you have already accomplished," was Grandma's reply, "and keep it where you can see it, to remind you that you should be proud of what you have already done."

After she died, as we all tried to find the words we wanted to share with people during her funeral service, we began to compile my beautiful grandmother's list of accomplishments. It was very cathartic for us to remember her words of advice and the many things that she did in her life to make us feel so proud of her and so loved by her.

Afterwards, I made a list of things I was proud to have accomplished in my own life. I listed big things like traveling, completing my university degree and writing the first draft of a novel, and I listed little things like learning to love my body—imperfections and all, falling in love, and having wonderful friends.

At first I felt a bit boastful and immodest, two things my grandmother certainly was not. But before long, my list made me feel a sense of accomplishment I had never had before. At times when I was feeling discouraged or disappointed in myself, I would remember my list and remember all of the things I had managed to do in my life. Then I would feel like my grandmother would be proud of me, and I even felt proud of myself.

I hung my list on my refrigerator and even added to it from time to time over the years. My friends liked to read it when they were over to visit, and a few of them created lists of their own.

I've moved several times since I began my list, but I still have it. Now I keep it in my wallet, and I've added "became a mother" to it. I still take it out now and then to remind myself of my successes and victories when I need some encouragement, and to find my personal strength again when I feel broken down. The self assurance that my list has given me has helped to guide me through some very difficult times since my beautiful grandmother died. I can't imagine a more valuable gift than what I've learned from her. My daughter didn't get to know my grandmother, but I gave her Grandma's name, and I have added "Teach Lilly about the list" to my list of things to do.

~Molly Cadigan

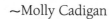

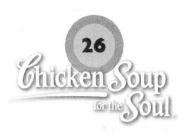

Fun

Attitude is a little thing that makes a big difference.
~Winston Churchill

One holiday season, way back in the 1980s, I was caught unprepared for the New Year. Somehow, I forgot to make a resolution, and didn't realize it until January 2nd, when my three office mates began discussing theirs. What to do?

I could have copped out. I could have said, "I don't make New Year's resolutions." But that would be a lie; I did make them. What's more, I liked them! I just... forgot.

Was it too late?

I don't know where the idea came from, but I opened up the Power Point program on my computer, printed out a sign in bold 32-point letters, and taped it to the wall in back of my desk. The sign read:

If it ain't fun, I ain't doing it.

When co-workers asked me my resolution, I pointed to the sign. Everyone laughed and a few double-entendres were muttered.

"Does that mean you're only going to do half your work?" one boss asked. "Because if I have to hire an assistant for you, we need to talk."

I worked for a small company where kidding and practical jokes were daily occurrences—often initiated by management. "An assistant would be great," I said. "She could give us all pedicures."

"I'll think about it."

A few days later the Sales Manager burst in. "I'm swamped. Clear your desk, you've got to help me. We've got a new promotion planned—well, not really planned, you're gonna get stuck with the planning stuff. A national contest... we're giving away T-shirts and sound systems. It'll run for three months. You need to schedule...." He stopped, catching sight of the sign behind me.

The Sales Manager tapped his pencil on his papers and turned away. He looked down the hall for a few seconds before flashing a huge smile at me. "You are going to love this! A national contest; this will be so much fun. You'll be talking about this for the rest of your life—you'll tell your grandchildren about it! You'll be meeting celebrities, writing radio promos...."

And so it went. Everyone who saw the sign reframed the tasks we did together. We discovered that ripping and separating six-part forms was actually cathartic and released tension. Running to the warehouse to check on orders could be great exercise. A phone call broke up a dull afternoon. Once, the boss brought in a six-pack of soda and announced that our weekly meetings would now start with belching contests.

If it ain't fun, I ain't doing it. Could I refuse the work that wasn't fun? Not without losing my job! I had to reset my own mind and find fun. It wasn't that hard; I liked my job to begin with. Invoices, shipping labels, customer service questions—all became, by wild (and sometimes twisted) leaps of the imagination, fun.

Not every story evolved into an anecdote, of course. Sometimes the fun was no more than an espresso or ice cream break when the work was done. My work didn't change, but my attitude did.

That resolution taught me that fun exists all around me, waiting to be found. Pain, drama, boredom, stress, and sadness are there too. We choose what to see and how to respond to it.

~Vickey Kalambakal

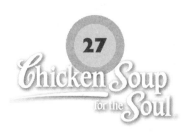

27

A Mother's Lesson

Don't wait to make your son a great man — make him a great boy.
~Author Unknown

While driving my eleven-year-old son, Bailey, to school, I was on my cell phone sharing my excitement about the wonderful stories we received for this book, *Chicken Soup for the Soul: My Resolution*. When I ended my call, Bailey asked if he could write a story. I was surprised by his request and asked if he had "resolved" to do something different in his life. How could he possibly have a resolution to make in his perfect world? His reply surprised me, as I had no idea that he even understood the concept of resolutions. He said, "I have resolved to be nicer to younger children and of course... make more goals during this soccer season."

My son is an only child, and the first boy born into a family that was accustomed to raising girls. He has grandparents who love to buy him "boy" toys and spoil him like crazy. My son is fortunate enough to have multiple gaming systems and more Hot Wheels cars and Lego sets than anyone he knows. Bailey has always been kind-hearted and generous with older kids and has never had a problem inviting them to join his fun. However, when it comes to younger kids, he falls short. He gets easily frustrated when they touch his Lego creations, play with his favorite Hot Wheels, or fail to understand how to play his video games.

My husband and I have many friends with younger children

who visit regularly. Each time before they arrive, we tell Bailey who is coming over and how we would appreciate it if he were patient and nice to the younger kids so that the adults can enjoy themselves. He starts out great, but as the night wears on his patience wears out. I found it interesting that our instructions did not fall on deaf ears and that he was voluntarily making an official resolution to include the younger kids in his play and show more patience.

As I continued to drive, I reflected on our conversation and realized that Bailey had actually been implementing his resolution all along without telling us or looking for praise. The last time our friend's son, Brayden, came over, Bailey invited him into his room and took out the tub of Legos. Instead of getting frustrated that Brayden was not building correctly, according to Bailey's standards, he allowed him to create his own version of an airplane or fort. When it was time to play video games, instead of telling Brayden he was too young to understand the concept, he gave him an "unplugged" controller and let Brayden believe he was in the middle of the battlefield right alongside Bailey.

As parents, we often feel as if our instructions or requests fall on deaf ears, but now I realize that my son has been listening all along. He is growing and maturing and striving to be a better person, just like all of us "resolving" adults. I dropped him off at school with love and admiration for my little boy who is becoming an amazing young man before my eyes.

~D'ette Corona

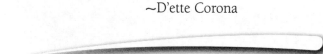

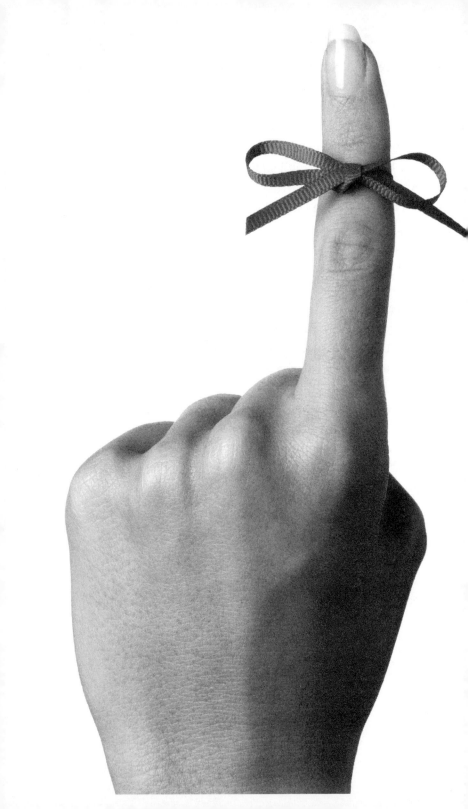

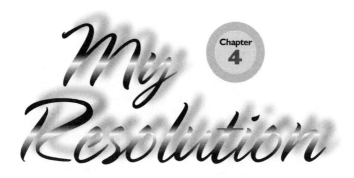

Chapter
4

Hello Body!

Inside some of us is a thin person struggling to get out,
but they can usually be sedated with a few pieces of chocolate cake.

~Author Unknown

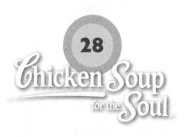

28

Baby Steps

Start now! Commit to be fit.
~Author Unknown

In January of 2002, my weight had hit an all-time high and I had fallen into the category of morbidly obese. I was in my early twenties, and I was supposed to be reveling in the prime of my life, but my health was fading rapidly. It would take me months to get over a simple cold, and only a few weeks later I would catch it again. There were other things, things I'd been too scared to tell anyone about. How I would wake up at night choking, because I'd stopped breathing in my sleep.

When a person struggles with an enormous amount of excess weight her entire life, it's easy for the subject of weight loss to be a taboo. I never wanted to tell anyone about my diet plans because I'd always ended up failing in my previous attempts, and I was ashamed. But this time I knew something had to be done; this time my life was depending on it.

I didn't even step on a scale on New Year's Day. I was too scared to read the numbers. Instead I eliminated any beverage from my diet that wasn't coffee or water. It was a baby step, but I knew every little bit helped. I also knew that if I could stick to this small change, the other changes I had planned would be easier to handle.

By the month of February, I'd confirmed to myself that I had the discipline I would need for the future. My pants were no longer cutting into my stomach, and it gave me the courage I needed to step on the scale. When the needle stopped spinning and landed on the number 240, I didn't allow myself to feel the usual guilt, self-pity, or sorrow. It was only a number, not a reflection of who I was, and I was determined to see that number disappear forever.

It took every scrap of leftover courage I could muster, but I began to tell people at work about my weight loss plans. Instead of a New Year's resolution, I told them it was just for the month of February; to see what I could accomplish in the shortest month of the year. To my surprise, others thought it was a great idea and jumped on the band wagon with me. I don't think I'll ever know if it was their way of gently encouraging me, or if they really loved the idea, but everybody was genuinely excited. They could all last twenty-eight days, and they loved that there was no pressure to continue afterwards. I was counting on my progress to be the motivational force to propel me forward.

I had an intense workout plan that I knew I could stick to for just a few short weeks. Three days a week I worked my entire body with free weights, and another three days a week I did cardiovascular workouts for my heart. On the days I felt lazy or reluctant, I would remind myself that it was only for a month, but more often were the days I looked forward to having that little bit of time to get my new-found energy out. I was surprised to learn that exercise was actually therapeutic.

When March finally came, I confronted the dreaded scale once again. To my surprise, I'd lost eighteen pounds! That week I went out and splurged on a few new shirts and a new pair of pants at a discount store. I didn't plan on being able to wear them for long, but wanting to look good and feel good about the progress I'd made was important. I knew that there would be times of discouragement ahead because I had a long path to travel down, but being reminded of how far I'd come was the biggest motivation I could think of.

After my intense workout of February, I took things a little easier, allowing myself time to adjust to the new weight. I hadn't wanted my body to feel starved from such an extreme loss in such a short period of time, and I also wanted my mind to know that I wasn't planning on denying myself forever. It's a precarious challenge trying to make the mind and body work together, and I didn't want to jeopardize any progress.

When I finally welcomed the next year, I was at least forty pounds lighter than I had been the previous year.

February rolled around again, and again I began my intense training session. My weight loss wasn't as significant as the first year, but it showed. By the end of the year, I'd lost a total of seventy pounds.

I still battle my weight every day, and I still have a few pounds that I would like to see disappear. I try not to rush myself though, and I remember that keeping the weight off is often just as difficult as losing it. Every February I celebrate my own personal New Year, and my extended lease on life. With patience and persistence, I am reminded of what baby steps can truly accomplish.

~Rebecca Degtjarjov

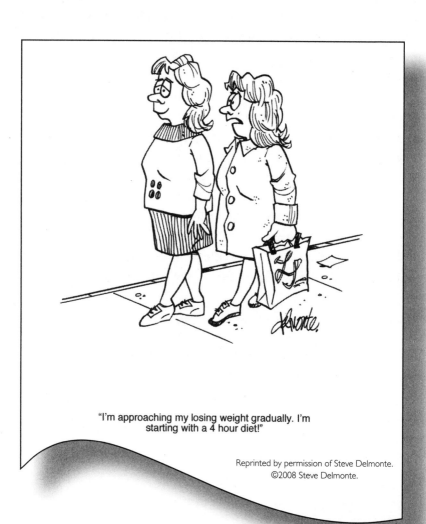

"I'm approaching my losing weight gradually. I'm starting with a 4 hour diet!"

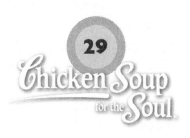

Because I Can!

You only live once; but if you live it right, once is enough.
~Adam Marshall

"What was I thinking? I must be some kind of fool!" I'm a fifty-three-year-old grandma crouched in an awkward position reminiscent of giving birth, perched before an open gate on a zip line platform high up in the hills above Maui's northwest coast, seemingly to plunge to my death. Again, I asked myself, "What was I thinking?"

Instead of living in the moment of joyous anticipation of flying like an eagle, I was experiencing some setbacks. I mean, coming in dead last in the walk up a hill while carrying a twenty-pound zip line cable trolley, and smelling like a goat, was mortifying and certainly didn't qualify as one of my finer moments. The brochure didn't say anything about that little hike. And the red welts growing exponentially on my shin from invisible flesh eating entities that burned, really burned, were certainly unattractive. Though, to be honest, the attack of the no-see-ems earned me the moniker of the group's "good sport" which I liked. But so far, this adventure wasn't fun — it was crazy. The near jarring of my teeth from their sockets on my first crash landing reminded me, this would not be good for me three more times.

I could have slept in, I could have had Sunday brunch with friends, and I could have taken a beautiful morning walk on one of Maui's incredible beaches. But Noooooooooooo; I had to fly through trees; I had to soar like an eagle; I had to stretch myself and do something I've never done before. Why?

Because I could! Because for the first time in my adult life, I met the weight requirements to go zip lining, and I had a point to prove—I CAN do anything I set my mind to. And if I can do it—so can any other overweight person on the planet who wants to change her life; hence, the childbirth crouch high atop a zip line.

I wasn't at my goal weight yet, but I gained admission into this activity through 93 pounds kicked to the curb. While I was working on losing the rest of my physical weight by incorporating activities like zip lining into my life, I was also working hard on losing the weight in my head. Leaving the world of obesity behind mentally was proving to be just as difficult as the weight loss itself, so I started thinking and acting like a thin person.

The wondrous roar of waterfalls and melodious songs of tropical birds drifted up to me from the treetops below, and I found it difficult to contain my emotions. I threw back my head and arms in a moment of euphoric weightlessness as I raced forty-five miles an hour down the mountain. "Whoo-hoo! Look at me! I'm flying!" My spirit soared! I left those 93 pounds behind and flew full speed toward my new life.

~Jeri Chrysong

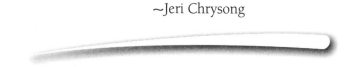

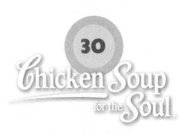

30

Un-Resolved

*The person who views himself at fifty the same as he did at twenty
has wasted thirty years of his life.*
~Muhammad Ali

Age sixty-three: Birthday resolutions: I will lose weight. I will exercise until my muscles are firm and my pot belly disappears. I will look like I did back when I weighed 100 pounds soaking wet and ate anything I wanted.

I knew it was possible. I knew it was easy. I'd done it before. Why not again?

So I joined a gym and went faithfully three days a week.

First came the equipment room. It was filled with tanned, well-muscled men, toned women dressed in miniature Spandex clothing. I heard the clank of metal against metal, but the only piece of equipment I recognized was the treadmill. Cautiously pushing the start button, I began walking. Nothing to it. But after a few days, boredom turned my brain to the consistency of spoiled peaches. I tried reading while walking, but the print in the magazines bounced with every step and I got so dizzy I was afraid I'd go flying off the end and land ungracefully in a sweatpants and T-shirt heap against the wall.

Maybe, I decided, classes would be better. Yoga. I became very good at lying on my back on my purple mat, palms up, relaxing. In fact, I was an excellent relaxer. It was all those other poses that made me decide I wasn't yoga material after all. The day I crouched on the floor, looked out from under my leg, and vaguely tried to put my foot somewhere over my shoulder, I knew it was time to move on.

I'd never tried belly dancing. It looked like fun. How hard could it be? I bought a pale blue scarf with hundreds of little coins sewn on it and tied it around my waist. The metal coins jingled happily as I positioned myself in the second row. The music played. I swayed. And then I watched the teacher's firm hips gyrate in directions my hips would never go. Not in a million years. I tried. The jingling, pale blue scarf I'd been so proud of slid slowly to the floor as I shimmied. It went in the car's trunk with my yoga mat.

Line dancing? I couldn't remember the steps if there were more than four. Cardio? My face turned red and I was left gasping for air.

Did my muscles become firm with all of this effort? They did not. They screamed and cramped if I so much as approached the gym, and revolted by keeping me awake at night.

I didn't lose weight, either. In fact, I gained two pounds.

And that's when I saw myself reflected in the window of the No-Longer-Petite Store, over near the mall. Windows don't lie. "No matter what you do, woman," it said, "you'll never look like you did forty years ago. Get real. Check it out. Hair turning gray. Sensible shoes. Square body. Think you're going to look twenty again? It ain't gonna happen."

And that's when the happy truth hit me like a runaway skateboard. I'm at a different stage in my life now. Oh, I can exercise for my health, but nothing will ever give me back the body of my youth. And if I'm able to diet, I still won't end up looking like a thin and sleek magazine model babe; I'll just be a bony old lady.

Me? An old lady? Hey, that's what I am! The thought was liberating. I smiled. I wanted to dance right there on the sidewalk, and even took a few quick steps.

I was finally free to be me. To do what I wanted. To forget about what people expected. And guess what? I realized I was already a terrific old lady. I had smile crinkles surrounding my eyes. I welcomed any adventure that might come my way. And I was equipped with enough padding to make a comfortable lap for grandchildren to climb into.

Age sixty-three and a half: Un-birthday resolution: I'll be what I am, live in the moment, and enjoy the ride. After all, that's what life's all about!

~Michele Ivy Davis

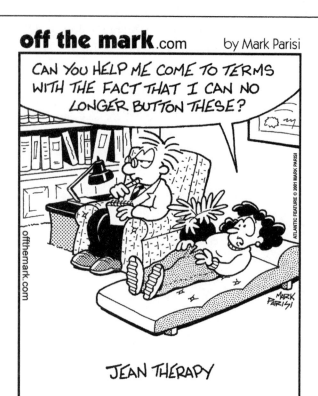

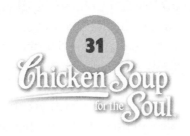

31

My Last Diet

Take charge! "I must do something" always solves more problems
than "Something must be done."
~Author Unknown

So far, it had been like any other speaking trip: decent flight, new city, nice hotel, my room service tab taken care of. Mmmm. Room service.

But shortly after I boarded my flight home, there was a glitch: after much concentration and effort—all the while trying to make the process look "normal"—I hadn't succeeded in buckling my seatbelt. How I'd come to hate this moment, when no matter how well I thought I'd camouflaged it, I had to acknowledge the reality of my belly. But the crisis usually passed and I conveniently forgot.

Now I was panic-stricken: Would I have to ask the flight attendant for help? Did they have extenders for people like me?

I sucked it in as best I could and gave it one more try. Click. A sigh of relief. But what about the next time?

Sigh and Surrender had been the name of the game for me for twenty years as I shifted up from petites to misses to what they politely call Woman—omitting the still silently screaming adjective Big/Abundant/and let's face it: FAT. As I continued to march my ponderous way up the clothes rack, at 22w I wondered what was to come: I was on the next-to-the-last size.

Today, after losing 90 pounds, I look back and see a spirit of defeat I can hardly believe was part of me—white flags everywhere!

Where did it start? Was it my obsessively-thin mother who wore only skintight 50s sheath dresses—a woman anorexic way back before the problem had a name? As a 5'5" teen weighing in at 135 pounds, I was hopelessly convinced that I was fat—I only had to look at my perfect mom to be reminded.

Was it the early sexual abuse which eventually led me to promiscuity, drugs and alcohol during my twenties and thirties? Was it my desire to become a good mother that led me to distance myself from my earlier social confusion by making myself as shapeless and unattractive as possible?

The answers to these questions are not as important as the fact that it wasn't until I started losing weight that I began asking: Why would a woman with several decades of life still ahead cripple herself, her family and her future by lugging around an extra hundred pounds?

For me, being fat—and, yes, I use the f-word because early on I decided honesty was the best policy—was not a victimless crime. With a husband and eight children still at home I was certainly not the wife and mother I could have/would have/should have been. As the excess inches peeled off, so did my denial. As my energy level increased, I came to grips with the fact that through the years I had become less and less involved in the things we had once loved: the outdoors, hiking, discovering new places. If forced past my reluctance to don a bathing suit, I sat glued to one spot until the ordeal was over.

Early on I felt the need to acknowledge the loss my obesity represented to my family. No matter their protestations—"We love you the way you are, Mommy!"—they were dealing with a mom twice the size she should have been with half the get-up-and-go.

I thought my family's acceptance meant unconditional love. Looking back ninety pounds lighter, I see it means something else: hopelessness and denial.

While my original resolution was shaped as a simple imperative—Lose Weight!—this was just one example of the unexpected insights and opportunities for growth that came with my sticking to it.

There was also letting go of my sense of entitlement. Since I was responsible for feeding my family—none of whom had a weight problem—I had to learn to handle food without sampling it myself. As I resisted the nagging impulse to bring my hand to my mouth, I could feel another layer of denial being stripped away. I had eaten more than I'd admitted to myself.

I resisted self-pity by imagining a broke bank teller who had to handle other people's money all day while struggling to pay his own bills. I fought my envy of those gifted with I-can-eat-and-eat-and-not-gain-weight metabolisms by thinking of my son Jonny who has Down syndrome and has to work a lot harder than others, yet who is consistently full of joy.

As I learned how much less I needed to eat to survive and thrive, I found the same true in other areas of my life. I found myself cleaning out closets and drawers—riding the downsizing trend. It seemed in every area of our family's life, I'd over-consumed: Too many clothes, toys, dishes, knickknacks.

As I lost my reluctance to let things go, I found a spirit of liberation that was as emotionally exhilarating as the new freedom which allowed me to sprint to the bus stop to meet my kids—without running out of breath at all.

At the doctor's office eighteen months later, when the nurse weighed my son in at ninety pounds—the exact amount I'd lost—I didn't know whether to laugh or cry. But it all became clear, as I imagined carrying him with me 24/7, how I'd burdened myself while trying to pretend my life was normal.

In fact, as I freed myself from excess weight, I found my imagination soaring as my mental energy was no longer consumed with denial of what had truly been my greatest limitation—a limitation I had to admit had been completely self-imposed.

I won't gloss over the grieving process I've had to deal with—for the loss of the years before my big resolution. But the smorgasbord of unexpected benefits—the emotional, intellectual, spiritual, and economic freedom I've gained from losing weight have made a profound difference on the rest of my life.

Today when I scrunch into my seat for a flight and pull that seat belt tight, my seatmate may wonder why the big smile. All I can say is that seatbelt means so much more to me. It's a reminder that all it takes to turn your life around is to finally say, "I've had enough." And in cases like mine, to learn to say it every day for the rest of your life.

~Barbara Curtis

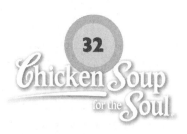

One Bite at a Time

One of the very nicest things about life is the way we must regularly stop whatever it is we are doing and devote our attention to eating.

~Luciano Pavarotti

For the past several years, with varying degrees of success, I've begun each January with the same two resolutions: lose weight and slow down my hectic pace of life.

Little did I know that the ability to achieve both resolutions would be connected to ten almonds.

After many attempts to lose weight, and with a history of yo-yo weight loss, I finally succeeded in moving the numbers on my bathroom scale down from the plateau that had plagued me. The magic solution wasn't so magical after all—a common-sense approach to eating sensibly and exercising regularly.

A loss of twenty-five pounds gave me reason to celebrate, at least until I hit the next plateau. This one lasted several months. Since I'm not, by nature, a patient person, the frustration from my most recent lack of progress carried over into other areas of my life.

Maybe I was missing something. I returned to the diet books. My newest diet plan included a mid-afternoon snack consisting of only ten almonds. It looked reasonable on the page... until my hunger pangs began to growl. Later that day, I didn't need a clock to tell me that it was time for the permitted afternoon munchies. I removed ten almonds from the jar and held them in the palm of my hand. The snack suddenly seemed paltry at best.

I popped several almonds into my mouth. They tasted good—I think! I was so hungry that I practically inhaled them. The first three nuts didn't make a dent in my appetite, so I gobbled the next four and then finished off what remained.

And then there were none.

It didn't take me long to retrieve the jar of almonds from the pantry. Ten nuts might be an adequate snack for a squirrel, but not for me! I devoured another handful before reluctantly placing the jar back on the shelf.

The next afternoon, I reached for my mid-afternoon snack once again. I dutifully counted out ten almonds. I lined them up on the counter and eyed them skeptically. Ten little soldiers all in a row.

Once more I popped a few into my mouth, repeating the action until I eliminated the line of almond soldiers.

I resisted the urge to reach for reinforcements. This was ridiculous. If the diet plan restricted my snack to ten almonds, then I should be able to accept the limitations.

The third afternoon, I counted out ten almonds, determined to make this work. This time I would do it right. I picked up the first almond and bit into it, slowly chewing and enjoying the flavor and texture. Then I picked up the next one. Once again I chewed slowly, savoring the light, nutty flavor. By the tenth almond, I realized that this was the first time I had slowed down long enough to truly enjoy what I had eaten. More importantly, it was enough.

As I changed the way I snacked, I realized that my eating habits had sabotaged my dieting efforts. With apologies to a particular brand of potato chips, not only could I not eat just one... I could not eat just one at a time. I would pop two or three chips into my mouth, justifying my behavior. After all, they weren't whole chips, they were broken pieces.

I soon became aware that these poor eating habits went beyond snacking. Even when I enjoyed eating sit-down meals with others, invariably I was the first one finished, having gobbled down my food and dutifully cleaned my plate.

I had to re-learn how to eat, to actually experience the taste of what I ate, instead of thoughtlessly shoveling food into my mouth. I began to eat my meals more slowly, making a conscious effort to enjoy the various colors, textures and flavors of each morsel: soft or crispy, tender or chewy, sweet or sour, salty or spicy. Eating more slowly enabled me to fill up more quickly, which meant I ate less but enjoyed it more. I learned to truly appreciate what I ate—one raisin at a time, one peanut at a time, one chip at a time. One bite at a time.

I soon discovered a surprising benefit, having nothing to do with dieting, but having everything to do with life.

For years I had complained about my hectic life. I spent most of my days running from one errand to the next, from one meeting to the next, and from one commitment to the next. And I prided myself on my ability to multi-task. Taking a telephone call while tracking my e-mail. Reading the newspaper while eating breakfast. Doing a load of laundry while cooking dinner. Balancing the checkbook while watching television.

I had forgotten what it felt like to do one thing at a time and do it well. Instead, I had resigned myself to doing several things simultaneously with mediocrity.

Those ten almonds taught me a better way. To truly savor each moment, I needed to concentrate on the task at hand, not the one coming later or tomorrow or next week.

The year is half over, and I've broken through my weight-loss plateau. The pounds are coming off again, slowly, but surely.

And I'm learning to live life... one precious bite at a time.

~Ava Pennington

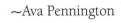

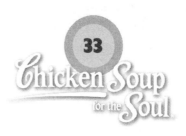

Shaping Up

*I have gained and lost the same ten pounds so many times over
and over again my cellulite must have déjà vu.*
~Jane Wagner

Staring at myself in the cruel light shining on the dressing room mirror, I said aloud, "I look pathetic." I meant every word of it. Without question, a good ten pounds had to come off—the same ten pounds that had appeared on every New Year's resolution list in recent memory.

I usually managed to take off the weight. I had plenty of practice and knew precisely how to adjust my diet in the kitchen, but the weight seemed to always creep back on when I wasn't looking. Something seemed to be missing and I knew what it was—exercise.

So, this year was going to be different. I resolved to pull out all the stops. I wanted to be toned and firmed and fit as a fiddle. I felt great when I discovered a woman's health club not far from home.

My first visit included embarrassing stuff, like recording vital statistics, my weight, and my body fat. I would begin classes designed to tone and firm my flab the following week.

Monday found me purchasing workout attire. I even found a gym bag with coordinating colors. My husband watched with a look that said, "Go ahead, but you'll fizzle out within a month." I deserved that look. Three years earlier, after my doctor recommended a good exercise program for my back, I had hired a professional trainer to come to my home and devise a customized workout for me. I was ecstatic about the possibilities and did everything she advised—for about six weeks.

"Never mind that," I told myself, "this time would be different."

At one o'clock, Wednesday afternoon, I marched into the gym; my spiffy bag flung across my shoulders in a way I hoped made me appear a veteran at working out.

Joining my fellow-flabbies on the exercise floor, I was pleasantly surprised to discover all shapes and sizes.

As the music started, an instructor named Kinsey, not weighing more than ninety pounds, stood before us and began barking orders.

"Okay! Are we ready?"

I was. At least, I thought so.

"Stand up nice and tall!" she yelled. "That's it! Let's warm up our shoulders and arms! Here we go! Roll 'em in! Take 'em out! Roll 'em in! And take 'em out! Great!"

Just about the time I mastered rolling 'em in and taking 'em out, the music's tempo shifted, and Kinsey yelled, "Okay! Let's warm up the upper back and those abdominal muscles!"

Oh, boy. I was short of breath already. If this was a mere warm-up, I smelled trouble.

"Keep those abdominals tight, ladies! Take it down! And pull it out! Beautiful! Take it down! And pull it out! Great! You feel it stretching?"

Not to worry. The leotard would never be the same.

"Stretch it out!" Kinsey screamed. "Use your legs now!"

Mine were trembling violently.

Kinsey was merciless. "Lunge!" she hollered, in perfect syncopation with the music. "Lunge! Two, three, four. Lunge! Two, three, four. Beautiful!"

I noticed Kinsey hadn't broken a sweat. To make matters worse, she was staring right at me.

"If you start to feel weak," she yelled, not missing a step, "take a little break." She smiled in my direction. "Side to side, now!" she screamed. "Come on, ladies! Push it back! Move those legs! Push it back! Keep that tummy tight!"

A couple of hours later, I dragged myself into the house and collapsed in a pile on the den floor. I now understood why exercise helped you lose weight: You were too tired to eat.

I still lay in a flaccid heap when my husband arrived home. "What happened to you?" he asked.

"Exercise," I moaned. "Call 911."

"I will make supper," he offered. I could only groan.

Later, as I trudged to the table, my face a picture of distress, my husband grinned.

"Are you making fun of me?" I asked, annoyed.

"No," he chuckled.

"So why are you laughing?"

"I am laughing at how silly you are."

I looked puzzled.

"There is nothing wrong with your body," he said. "and you aren't even close to fat." He patted my shoulder reassuringly.

As we said grace, I kept my head bowed a moment longer. I wanted to say special thanks for a man who not only knew how to cook, but how to stay out of hot water, as well.

~Dayle Allen Shockley

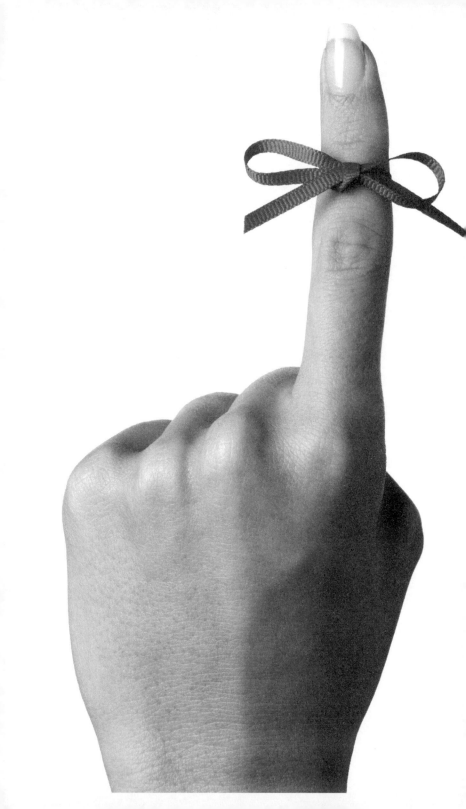

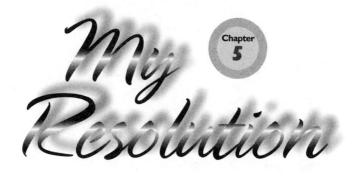

Chapter
5

I'm Worth It

Learn to... be what you are, and learn to resign with a good grace all that you are not.

~Henri Frederic Amiel

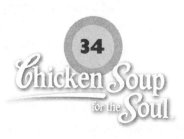

The Baggy Sweatsuit Monster

Be beautiful if you can, wise if you want to, but respect yourself—
that is essential.
~Anna Gould

I pushed my grocery cart through the wide aisles. It was making a horrible squeaking noise. I decided to ignore it and hoped that no one else noticed. The last thing I wanted to do was draw attention to myself. I continued walking, passing other women who were filling clear plastic bags with vegetables and fruits. I went straight to the cookie aisle. My boys were quarreling over what kind of cereal we should buy while I tried to decide between the chocolate chip cookies with the cream center or chocolate stripe graham cookies.

All of a sudden a man, a handsome man, about 6'1" turned down the aisle and began to push his cart in my direction. A flood of sweat beaded on my face and trickled down my sides. I looked a mess. I looked anything but normal. You see, I didn't bother to put any effort into my appearance before going to the store. Why should I? Would anyone notice if I fixed my hair or put on make-up? You see, no matter how much time you put into selecting your outfit or dolling yourself up, when you weigh 250 pounds, no one ever compliments your appearance. I quickly walked, almost ran from the aisle.

When I first got married in 2000, I was a hot little thing. The key word being "little." No I wasn't a size two and could probably even be considered plump by some standards, but at 5'7" and 175 pounds. I was looking better than I had in years, maybe ever! I had heard many stories of housewives who, once the kids come, completely let themselves go. I vowed I wouldn't ruin my marriage like that. I'd always try to look my best even when I didn't plan on leaving my house that day. I promised myself that if I ever became a parent, I would never become the "Baggy Sweatsuit Monster."

I managed to keep my word for a whole year, but shortly after my first child was born, I decided I wanted to resign my womanhood. Who could blame me? I became a day care provider, chauffeur, counselor, chef, nurse, entertainer, personal stylist, and educator all at once. My entire life now centered on motherhood. I had absolutely no interest in appearing attractive to anyone. I re-designed my appearance to accommodate my own sense of convenience. I stopped wearing make-up, perfume, and jewelry. I bought jeans with the elastic band on them. I didn't even shave my legs.

Becoming a parent brought about many changes for me. But there was one constant in my life — food. Over time, food had become more than just something to eat; food was my comfort. Nothing calmed my anxieties like a big bowl of double chocolate chunk ice cream, and it was always available. My waistline expanded over the years as my self-esteem, my concerns for my marriage, and my health all diminished.

One day I was strolling down the frozen dessert aisle when I caught a glimpse of myself in the freezer case. I wasn't at all prepared for what was looking at me. There she was, staring back at me in the glass, the "Baggy Sweatsuit Monster." I knew I had put on some weight, but I didn't know I had ballooned from fit to flab over the course of seven years! The thirty-three year old, once beauty now fatty, had obviously let herself go. How did I let this happen? Suddenly my anxieties grew. They proved to be too much for even the chocolate ice cream.

Later that night, I sat on my bed and gazed at a well-polished wedding picture of my husband and me. You see, it was all I had as proof that I was once beautiful. My pen began to stream across the pages of my journal. Through tears of frustration and anger, I wrote as if my life depended on it. I exhaled a flow of sorrow, guilt and sadness. When I finished, I had a plan; one I call "Thirty-five before Thirty-five." I had a list of things I was determined to accomplish before turning thirty-five years old. It was a good plan, but I knew the only way to make it happen was to learn to love myself.

Included on my list was learning to smile a little each day, learning to laugh sometimes, learning to look in the mirror and love who I see... flaws and all.

I will love myself enough to take care of myself—to make conscious choices about what I put in and on my body.

In learning to love myself, I will learn that self-pampering does not equal selfishness. There's no harm in giving myself the respect that I deserve. Besides, in taking some "me" time, I set a good example for my children. If my body and mind are weakened from neglect, I can't be the supportive mother I so desperately want to be.

Now I discover a way to love and pamper myself everyday, whether it's by painting my toes, styling my hair, getting a facial, buying a new lotion, spending an afternoon at a spa, trying a new eye shadow or putting on lipstick for a quick errand to the grocery store.

Today, before going grocery shopping, I gazed in the mirror. I saw a drastic difference from what appeared months ago in the freezer case. The soft brush of magenta and rose eye shadow brought out the sparkle in my eye. My cascading black hair flowed onto my shiny bare shoulders. I looked like a new person. No, I'm still not a size two and am still considered plump by most standards, but the ugly monster is gone, and she's not welcome back.

~Annita Hammonds

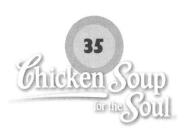

Learning to
Make a Resolution

We must be willing to get rid of the life we've planned,
so as to have the life that is waiting for us.
~Joseph Campbell

It was December 31st at 11:30 P.M. I had ducked into the washroom to check my make-up and take a breather. Once again, I had been invited to a party of married couples and those soon-to-be married. Friends and family, but nonetheless still the only awkwardly single, well—divorced and single woman in the room. I did look good though in my little black dress and perfect pumps but really, who was here to notice except my best buddies; my sisters. Their compliments were sweet at the beginning of the evening, and appreciated, but now as I was fast approaching the hour of couples kissing in the New Year those compliments were giving me little solace.

I knew that I would have to face bringing in another year by kissing either the dog or, if I were lucky, I could sneak upstairs to my sleeping nephew and peck his cheek while he lay in his crib. The kissing part was uncomfortable, but really not the worst part of it all. Oh no, that would have to be the proverbial decision to come up with some resolution that I would be able to follow through with for once.

I stared in the mirror for a short time and then decided I should rejoin the others or, heaven forbid, miss out on the whole ritualistic display of affection. But the thoughts continued to cross my mind and then, like a light, it hit me.

This was going to be my year. I was going to make everything happen and why shouldn't I? I would lose those pesky fifteen pounds, eat healthful meals, and start working out with a vengeance. I would meet Mr. Right and we would happily fall into blissful and absolute love within moments of seeing each other across a crowded room. Oh, how romantic! I would write my bestselling novel and be swooped into a book tour across Europe and of course, meet Robert De Niro who was set to play the lead in the film version.

My gosh, my world would be terrific. Never mind these practical and predictable married types and their world of responsibilities, potluck dinners, school plays and bickering over where to put the new sofa. I was going to be fabulous and live a fabulous life and that's all there was to it. What a stupendous dream! And that's exactly what it was — a dream.

I guess no one can predict what's going to happen to them in any given year. I could not have predicted that a colleague would have chosen death over life that New Year's Eve. I couldn't have predicted that in February, I would meet a man who would invite me to an impromptu vacation in Las Vegas, only to be involved in a car crash that killed his best friend hours before we were set to leave. I couldn't have predicted that my four-year-old niece would be diagnosed with cancer, along with my father, and that my mother would battle her cancer again for a second time.

I could not have predicted the challenge of my personal relationships and my decision to end some friendships because they were no longer healthy for me. I could not have predicted the loneliness that came at the end of the year. I couldn't have predicted any of it. But then again, I don't think I could have predicted the lessons I learned either.

I learned that each year brings new hope for things to come and problems are never so big that death should ever be the only answer. I learned that plans change and we need to be flexible, and when I can help someone who has experienced a loss, I want to do it because it makes me feel good to help. I learned to rejoice over the little things and indulge in the simple things, such as spending time with family and friends. I learned that a four year old has more strength than most grown-ups and resilience is indeed a gift. I learned that it's okay to let go of those who don't make us feel good about ourselves, and it's okay to feel lonely every now and then; we're human. And I learned that life is not about predicting what will happen next, but about learning from the moments that will make up the next moments.

It's December 31st again, exactly 11:30P.M., and once again I'm going to make a resolution for the New Year to come. Nothing grandiose, just this: this year I will appreciate the experiences that I am given and hope that through the months to come I will learn a little something about myself, my world, and my life that may just make it a little better than it was before.

~Deborah Batt

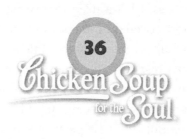

Less Grief, More Green

We must embrace pain and burn it as fuel for our journey.
~Kenji Miyazawa

As the new year dawned, I was at one of the lowest points of my life. In March, my beloved sister Sherry died. My dear friend Bob died in August. Even my sweet dog Molly died that November. In addition, my husband Alan's medical condition was getting progressively worse. Alan had a massive heart attack and cardiac arrest five years earlier that left him with a severe brain injury from lack of oxygen. The brain injury led to dementia and Parkinson's disease. Although Alan excelled at being his best self, he needed and deserved my love and care around the clock.

Living in this world of illness, grief, and loss left me wrung out physically, emotionally and spiritually. I knew I needed to replenish my energy and outlook even as I rode the tides of ongoing grief.

Nature has always been a source of healing, reflection, and rejuvenation for me. My favorite sanctuary is the Arnold Arboretum of Harvard University in Boston, a marvelous 265-acre living museum of trees from all over the world. Inside the Arboretum gates, visitors can explore meadows, hills, and miles of paths away from the city streets and rushing traffic.

One afternoon, I sat in a nook formed by the spreading roots of a copper beech tree. Protected by a generous mantle of boughs, I let my mind roam over the sorrows and happier occasions of the past year. After so much loss, I felt a need to give myself to the turning of seasons—the snow-covered dormancy of winter, followed by the unfolding of new life in spring. I wanted time away from the worry and constant, serious responsibility that every caregiver knows so well. I decided to find new ways to get involved with nature as one way of bringing a restorative balance to my life. As I walked home, my New Year's resolution took shape in my mind. My resolution became "Less grief, more green."

"Less grief, more green" was my rallying motto and I looked for ways to put it in action. I joined the Arnold Arboretum training program for volunteer school field guides. The field guides provide outdoor learning experiences for Boston public school students in grades three to five. As a lifelong urban dweller, I welcomed the chance to introduce children to nature as a source of pleasure and curiosity for years to come.

In order to meet the volunteer commitment, I had to deepen my trust, take some risks and make some changes. Instead of being home with Alan all the time, I had to entrust more of his care to our dedicated and competent home health aide. This was a big transition, but Alan, a scientist and teacher, supported the idea as long as I brought home what I was learning to share with him.

Nancy, the program director, provided guides with several bountiful days of training. I dived into the spring curriculum on pollination. The thick notebook brimmed with information and diagrams about how flowers and tree flowers bud, bloom, and produce the seeds that assure that the species will continue.

While in training, I relished being a student again, instead of the expert I had to be to manage Alan's care. In the circle of guides, who ranged from college students and mothers to retired plant experts, illness was not a distraction or topic of conversation. Instead we asked each other, "Which azalea bushes have the most pollen this week?" and "How do I explain the male and female flower parts to fourth-grade boys without making them snicker?"

A morning spent dissecting daffodils under a microscope made me happier and more energetic than I'd felt in months. Back at home

I set up a selection of flowers and fruits on the kitchen table and gave Alan a magnifying glass to identify the stamen, pistols, and ovules. He and Uche, our Nigerian aide, were enthusiastic students. "Demonstrations are the best part of science," said Alan, a retired physics professor.

After weeks of training, it was time to guide. A field trip to the Arnold Arboretum gives students a day full of information, excitement, and surprises. When sixty third-graders piled off the yellow school bus for the "Flowers Change" class, we gathered into small groups in the lecture hall to look at buttercups with a hand lens and practice words for the parts.

The kids watched an old-fashioned movie reel about the life cycle of cherry blossoms. They loved the ending when the mother bird feeds her babies the ripe cherry fruit and we talk about how birds spread cherry seeds.

Then the students built a model flower, acting out the roles of the stamen, pistol, and petals. The child manning the bee puppet hammed it up as he buzzed in to gather pollen and deposit it firmly on the head of the student playing the sticky stigma.

Finally the teams of junior scientists swarmed the Arboretum armed with hand lenses, fuzzy black pipe cleaners to gather pollen, and the most important tools of all—their senses. As we moved from the spectacular Elizabeth magnolias to the tulip poplar trees and katsura dogwoods, the kids collected colorful specimens and drew the stages of a flower. I encouraged the students to stoke the ridged bark of an oak tree, sniff skunk cabbage, and pause to listen to birdsong and spring peepers. On a super-good day they might meet Bertha, the ancient snapping turtle meandering to the pond to lay her eggs.

Throughout my first spring of practicing "less grief, more green," my senses came alive and expanded. My self-image tenderly bloomed beyond being a wounded caregiver to being a guide in my sanctuary. I moved beyond wonder and astonishment about nature to a better understanding. I learned about the workings of a child's mind along with the workings of trees and flowers.

Although I continued to grieve, those days spent under blue

skies observing the cycles of life brought me joy and gave me a connection to the world beyond myself and my family.

I went on to be a proud and enthusiastic Arnold Arboretum field guide for four seasons. I still carry all that understanding and curiosity about what I don't know each time I'm out in nature. And I still look at a tulip through the eyes of a third-grader.

~Janet M. Cromer

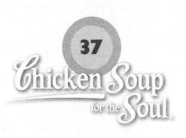

The Best Mother's Day Present I Never Got

*Things turn out best for the people who
make the best out of the way things turn out.*
~Art Linkletter

My resolution didn't start out in the traditional sense, as a personal resolve made at the threshold of the New Year. No, mine came about much more covertly—stealthily camouflaged in the guise of ingratitude and sullenness.

Two years ago—Mother's Day 2006—my life changed, and I owe it all to the best present I never got.

Benchmark events change a woman's life forever—graduating, getting married, having a child—the "biggie" events in many women's lives. But events like those are often anticipated and foreseen. What made Mother's Day 2006 so very different for me was that I did not immediately recognize the true transformative nature of the life-changing gift that had been bestowed upon me.

•••

The day started out simply enough. Sleeping in on a lazy Sunday morning, I awoke about 8:00 A.M. with the quasi-expectation of being roused by the sounds of my sons and my husband sweeping into the room, carrying a tray brimming with goodies for a leisurely and luxurious breakfast in bed.

When that didn't happen, I got up, got dressed and then went downstairs, expecting a "SURPRISE!" or at least a heartfelt "Happy Mother's Day!" Again... nothing. Just two kids plopped in front of the TV and my husband on the computer.

The day continued to unfold uneventfully, and while I was not waiting with bated breath for a present or mom-centric celebration, I did have the minimal expectation of at least being acknowledged, and perhaps even thanked with a few words of gratitude. Something along the lines of, "Thanks for giving me life and bringing me into this world, and for providing for my every need and the majority of my wants. Thank you for saying 'no' to me for my own good, even when I 'hate' you for it and would really like you to say 'yes,' knowing full well it would probably be to my own detriment."

Okay, nothing quite that self-aware or mature, but at least a token "Thanks Mom, I love you!" Something simple to complete my family's own little Hallmark moment.

The day wore on with nary a word about the significance of the day. "Aha! They must be planning a stealth dinner out somewhere," I told myself. Dinnertime rolled around and with no sign of going out, I plopped some frozen enchiladas into the oven (its temperature assuredly Siberian compared to my boiling and seething inside).

• • •

That's it! How dare they? I cannot believe they didn't do anything for me, and that the entire day went by with not so much as a "Happy Mother's Day, Mom!" Okay. I get it. You all think it's all about you, and that I am just some extraneous presence put in this household to serve you all. Well, I'll show you! From now on, I am putting all of you and your needs on the back burner and tending to MY wants, MY needs and MY desires first!

When I finished ranting my stream-of-consciousness soliloquy, I resolved to start making time for me, and to pursue my long-neglected passions and talents—those I'd subjugated to the maternal and marital duties of taking care of my family. I logged onto the Internet and enrolled in the online writing course I'd had my eye on but never had enough time to take when I was so terribly busy putting my family first and me last.

Six weeks went by, and I learned so much from the class and my wonderful instructor that I succeeded in selling my first article before the course was over. Bolstered by this success, I timidly approached my local town paper, inquiring if they might be in need of a freelance writer to cover local topics. Lo and behold, they said yes, and I was now being published weekly and thus further along on a life's journey I never planned to take.

I took more writing classes, and started getting more articles accepted for publication. After the third article, from a national periodical, my husband looked at me one day and said, "You're really a writer!" Something about those words solidified my resolve and made me say, "Yes! This is my new profession!" It wasn't a hobby, or something I did in my spare time. His words cemented the fact that writing was now my career—a business that I made time for, and pursued with passion.

• • •

The dictionary defines "serendipity" as a natural gift for making useful discoveries by accident. I look back on Mother's Day 2006 now, not with anger or resentment, but with celebration and joy. I see it as the year when I was certain that I got "nothing," but instead got "everything."

I see now the great bounty I received—a gift far greater than could ever be found on a store shelf or a restaurant menu. Mother's Day 2006 brought to me a gift that until that day I had never even imagined—a new career, a renewed passion, and an opportunity to pursue my love of learning (and get paid!). A chance to commune with my fellow man, shape viewpoints and most importantly... to touch lives.

All of these things came not so much from my children, but from within myself. I look back and reflect that I was the only one holding me back from following my dreams and passion. I had been so busy doing for my family that I had let a part of me wither and waste away inside.

Resentful of that day's events, I could have easily wallowed in self-pity. Instead, I chose to make proverbial lemonade from lemons, and to crawl through the window God opened once He shut the door. I chose happiness over resentment, and opted to look for it within myself instead of seeking and depending on it from others.

I can laugh now, and fondly recall that the best Mother's Day gift I never got was one of the best presents my kids could ever have "given" me. I appreciate even more, however, that heeding that lesson was the greatest gift I could ever have given myself.

~Mary Hay Davis

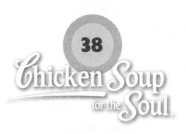

Just a Small New Year's Resolution

*Only those who will risk going too far
can possibly find out how far one can go.*
~T.S. Eliot

I sit in the high school auditorium and watch my youngest, Meagan, receive her diploma. The blue and yellow cords over her red gown testify to the awards she won and the excellent work she did in school. I think of her bright smile just a few days ago, when she received her scholarship award from the university of her choice.

Her older brother holds a degree in physics and computers, one sister is an engineer, and two other sisters are planning to attend evening classes at colleges near them. And to think all of this came about because of one simple, even selfish, New Year's resolution I had made many years ago!

That New Year's Eve, I returned to the living room from tucking the first two of my children into bed.

"I've decided on my New Year's resolution," my husband said, looking up from watching the New Year's celebration on TV. "I'm going to save for my pilot lessons. If I don't start now, I'll never achieve my dream of flying a plane some day."

"Good for you," I answered. "But what about me? I'm stuck

with the kids all day. It's not that I don't enjoy being a mother, but sometimes I wish I could do something for myself, too."

"Why don't you?" Gary suggested. "I'm sure you can think of something to do away from home." His attention returned to the show.

I sat down next to him, my eyes on the TV, and my thoughts about three thousand miles away. I could take an English class at the nearby college. That way, I'd get out of the house and learn something useful. And maybe I could improve my accent, so people would understand me better. After all, I'd come to the United States with my American husband only four years ago.

I grew up in post WWII Germany. At fourteen, after eight years of school, my mother sent me to work in a factory to support her and my five siblings. But even then I wanted more. I joined an American Christian church, and with the encouragement of my new friends, attended evening classes to learn English.

And now here I was, cut off from my family, mostly enjoying being a mother. But sometimes I wanted more. After all, I rationalized, if I take a class again, it wouldn't just benefit me; my children would have an advantage, too.

"You're right," I said. "I'll see if the college will allow me to take an English class. Just one class won't keep me away from the kids too long."

"Give it a try," my husband said. "I'm sure you'll do well."

But in my heart, I wondered. Taking a college class would be different from night classes learning English. I didn't know if I had the stuff to succeed in a university setting.

By the time classes started again, I realized I was expecting baby number three, so, half relieved and half disappointed, I postponed my resolution.

One day in March, after I'd put the kids down and finished cleaning up the supper dishes, my husband called to me from the living room, "I found a teacher."

Guilt made me almost drop the glass in my hand. "What teacher?" I yelled back.

"A pilot, licensed to teach flying."

"Oh." He wasn't talking about me, after all. Not everybody sticks to their New Year's resolution, I thought as I put away the last glass and then plopped onto the sofa next to him.

"What about your resolution?" he challenged me. "Have you signed up yet at the college?"

I shook my head. "I'm pregnant, you know."

"That shouldn't keep you from going back to school. If you sign up now, you could take the spring semester and be done in plenty of time before the baby comes."

I realized Gary was right. The worst that could happen would be that I'd drop the class again. I thought of the never-ending tasks at home, cooking three meals every day, a job I didn't really enjoy, chasing after Marja, the two year old, until I was exhausted, helping Dennis with homework, cleaning floors and washing dishes, wiping noses and changing diapers, and the prospect of soon having one more little life dependent on me. I knew I needed to do something for myself.

The next day, after dropping Dennis off at kindergarten, I took little Marja and we went to see the registrar at the college. I asked to be admitted to English 101 and told him I had the money ready. He made me fill out some papers. When he read them, he shook his head at my lack of a high school certificate.

"Okay," he finally said. "Try English 101. If you do well, you can keep taking classes."

I smiled as I returned to my car with a lighter heart.

A friend down the road babysat Marja three times a week while I attended class. I loved discovering the different styles of writing essays and trying my hand at them. At home, when I was busy with some routine task, in my head I went over what I had leaned that day, and in the evenings, instead of watching TV with Gary, I sat at the table doing my homework.

I walked away from that first class with an A+.

After Daniel was born, I took English 102 and 103, and then put my education on hold while my fourth child Marit, came along. Two years later, even though I was expecting again, I knew I had to return to school. This time I took three classes at a time and paid a babysitter with the money I made typing term papers for other students. Our home wasn't as clean as it used to be and the older children helped cook, but I was happier, and my kids were proud of their mom, who also went to school, just like they did.

Two years later the sixth child was on the way, but by that time my marriage had become rocky, and my need to have an education was strong. I finished finals for my second-to-last semester the day before Meagan was born, and I took her with me to classes as I finished my AA in English and Foreign Languages.

Half a year later, I separated from Gary and moved with my six children to Cedar City, where I attended the university full-time. I divorced my husband a year before I earned my BA in German, English, and Spanish, and a teaching certificate.

I taught high school for three years, and then I returned to the university for a Master's in Language Acquisition. Again, my children and I went to school together. I remember getting special permission from a professor during summer semester to bring little Meagan along with me to a class.

Now, as I sit in the auditorium, watching Meagan get ready for the university, I realize the impact of the New Year's resolution I made so long ago. Because I followed through on that resolution, education has changed not just my life, but the futures of all my children.

~Sonja Herbert

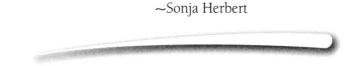

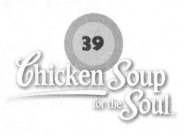

No

*Sometimes the most important thing in a whole day is
the rest we take between two deep breaths.*
~Etty Hillesum

It was a warm winter day and I remember wearing a short-sleeved red checkered blouse with my favorite blue skirt. Suddenly though, I felt a chill and I froze.

It was at a community meeting of women. I was comfortable as we visited and shared stories. And then, it happened. The hostess handed us each a paper and pencil and asked us to write down our New Year's resolution.

My pencil wouldn't write. Those around me smiled and wrote non-stop. I knew my friend to my left was writing about the new diet she was going to go on the first of the year. My friend to the right had to be writing about making more money in her job, as that was always her primary focus. Someone across the room was chuckling out loud as she described the man of her dreams who she was determined to find in the coming year.

I was blank. Blank and confused. I thought about my everyday life. I am content. Sometimes I am really tired and often wish there were more minutes in a day. But, don't most of us think those things? I am happy in my relationships. I love my job and my family and friends. I work out and feel fit. I volunteer in the schools, in the community and for many organizations. I am always there when someone needs me for carpool, an emergency, or to run an errand. Wow! What to do?

Others were folding their resolutions in half once and then again. The crackly sound of the paper folding annoyed me as my page was still empty. Everyone smiled as they placed their well-chosen words into a basket. Then they discussed openly and happily how the new year would change them. "For the better" was the agreement by all and a toast was made with sparkling cider. I wanted to be in on the toast.

My face turning red to match my shirt, I knew I had to write something. This same group of women vowed to look at these resolutions at the same party, same place, same time... next year. So in a rush I wrote something down, folded it and folded it again, and put it in the basket.

"Say no." That was all I inscribed on my resolution.

That was the best resolution I have ever made. And, I kept it! I realized on that warm winter day that I had become too busy doing for everyone else. I believe in volunteering and reaching out to help others. That is a gift I love to give. However, listening to the giggles and busy chatter about other women's daily lives, I heard the word "No" in my mind. I realized that I had stopped reading books, watching my favorite shows on television, baking fresh bread, or sitting on the couch relaxing. I resolved that I could still give to others, lead my busy fulfilling life, and also save time for me.

Each woman left with a colorful sparkly hat to wear on New Year's Eve and a hug for happiness in the New Year. I left feeling heavy, and wondering what they would think of me in one year when the paper with my brief words was unfolded.

On the way home, enjoying the birds singing and observing the colorful trees lining the street, I realized that it didn't matter. What mattered was, for once, me taking care of me. I even said it out loud, "I need to take care of me!" I never told anyone this before, but that New Year's resolution began even before the hands on the clock ever got to midnight for the New Year. When I got home, I brewed a cup of my favorite herbal tea, turned on the television, and turned on the answering machine.

I learned something that December day. Writing my resolution truly opened my eyes. I actually asked myself questions out loud: "Where had I been? What was I thinking?" I reflected back on being a child and always hearing my grandparents saying, "Life is too short." They are no longer here to know the impact they made on my most meaningful New Year's resolution. I never knew a New Year's resolution could work out and come true. Mine did, I think about it every year.

~Gail Small

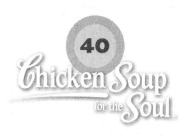

My Picture-Perfect New Year's Resolution

A happy person is not a person in a certain set of circumstances,
but rather a person with a certain set of attitudes.
~Hugh Downs

I never make resolutions. Every December 31st, at the stroke of midnight, my mind usually wanders from the resolution-making task at hand and is more concerned with why I'm not at a fabulous confetti-filled party somewhere, wearing a cocktail dress, and talking to a dashing gentleman (who might even have an accent). I mean, will all of my photo albums consist of consecutive New Year's Eves with me in my sweats, covered in cat hair, eating leftovers, with a distant glimmer of hope in my eye? Seriously? All I want is one, just one; fantastic picture to hang on my wall so all the world can see what an exciting and enviable life I lead—is that too much to ask? Not that I have anything against Dick Clark. He's a great date, and he always shows up.

One year, all of this sullen introspection got me to thinking about expectations. Why did I feel the pressure to have a picture-perfect New Year's Eve? Why did I care if people thought my life was exciting? Probably the same reason I felt like I should be settled in a career and married with three kids already. Throughout most of my life, I had deviated from the norm; somehow, I still felt it necessary to make apologies and excuses for my decisions.

But, why? Where was this desperate need to please coming

from? I had traveled the world, owned my own business, bought my first home, and started fulfilling my dream of writing all before the age of twenty-five. So what did I have to apologize for? Well, as previously stated, I was still single and indecisive about my career, which for a woman of my age was not considered "the norm." (Dear me, whatever shall they say at the class reunion?)

Then, suddenly, as I was about to ring in the new year by doing a load of laundry, an epiphany shone down from the heavens. It was a lightning bolt of realization. For my very first resolution, I was going to resolve not to care. Not to care about anyone's expectations but my own and to make no apologies for it. After all, I had gone wherever the road had taken me, and it had taken me to a lot of fabulous places—places I never would have been able to go if I had "settled down" already. Not to mention, I'd probably be starring in *Desperate Housewives* or making an appearance on *Divorce Court*.

And as far as my career went, being indecisive was just being honest. I couldn't change who I was just because I didn't fit into the social norm. At least I wasn't going to watch my life go by as I punched the clock at a job I hated, in order to climb a very shaky and uninteresting corporate ladder. No thanks! If I didn't try out my options, I would never discover my passions. And don't we all want to do something we feel passionate about?

Of course, these were all great thoughts, but actually incorporating them into my everyday thinking process would be a whole other story.... So, was I able to rise to the challenge of my very first resolution?

Well, let's just say that I have made the choice to be okay. Okay with my singlehood and my ever-changing career path, and okay that others might not be okay with it. I think that is the most important ingredient. And every New Year's Eve, I make sure to clear my schedule, dress up in my ugliest sweats, eat some delicious leftovers, and relax with my cat. Then as I tune in to watch the rest of the world create a picture-perfect New Year's, I glance at the photos on my own wall and think, "What a beautiful year it has been."

~Britteny Elrick

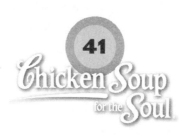

41

Can I Really Do This?

If you hear a voice within you say
"you cannot paint," then by all means paint,
and that voice will be silenced.
~Vincent Van Gogh

I am not giving up chocolate or martinis for my resolution. Or even chocolate martinis! But I am giving up something. And let me tell you, it's been hard. I mean, it's been really, really difficult. I am giving up being so hard on myself. I had no IDEA what a challenge that would be!

It's been a tough few days so far. No longer can I get upset if my hair doesn't look right, nor can I ask my husband if my behind looks too big in my jeans. I can't call myself an "idiot" for missing my exit, nor can I berate myself for having a messy closet. (And it does look like a tornado swept through it.)

My challenge is to be nice to myself. My goodness—was I ever self-programmed! Are you programmed to talk badly to yourself or to put yourself down? Do you tell yourself that you are stupid, old or klutzy—or too fat, too skinny, too tall or too short? My goal is to feel one hundred percent comfortable in my skin.

It's not all about my looks either. I can't be hard on myself if I make a mistake at work, if I burn the roast (I mean charred!) or make lumpy mashed potatoes. I can't chew myself out if I forget to mail my credit card bill (sorry, honey) or lose (misplace?) my car keys yet one more time.

I had no idea what a "hobby" my self-deprecation was! No longer can I glance sidelong into a grocery store window and compare myself to one of the Munchkins in *The Wizard of Oz*. (Remember the fat one in the green suit?)

Self-love is attainable—but first we have to, as Dr. Phil says, "Change our inner dialogue." Boy, that is not easy, is it? I'm not used to patting myself on the back—or looking into the mirror and thinking I look great! I'm not used to admitting to myself that yeah, dinner did taste pretty good tonight—I can really make a killer meatloaf. I'm not used to being thankful when I arrive at an appointment on time and in one piece and didn't yell at even one other car.

It's only been a few days. I am hoping that I can change my habits for good.... I keep smiling and telling myself that I am fine just the way I am, thank you!

~Karen Kelly

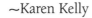

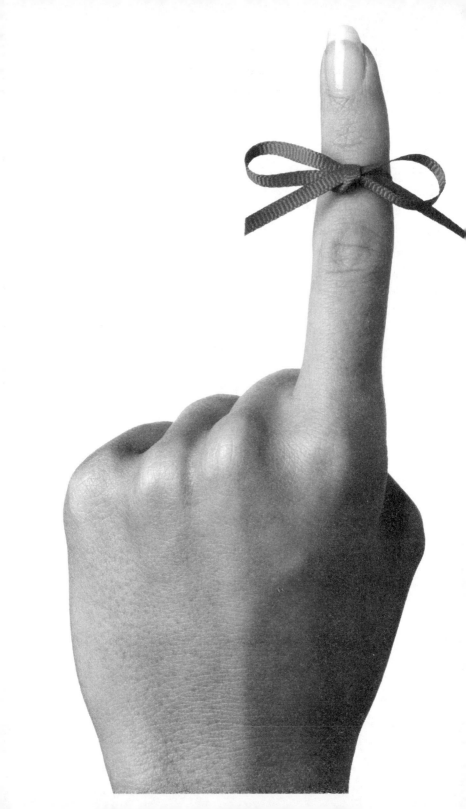

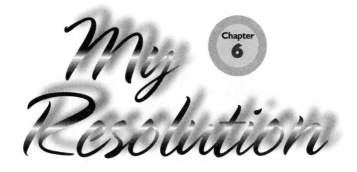

Chapter 6

Simple Pleasures

Slow down and everything you are chasing will come around and catch you.

~John De Paola

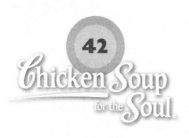

42

Confessions of a Morning Person

I love the sweet smell of dawn—
our unique daily opportunity to smell time,
to smell opportunity—
each morning being, a new beginning.
~Emme Woodhull-Bäche

t happened again today. I found myself apologizing to someone for being too perky in the morning. It wasn't even that early. I called a client at 9:00 A.M.—after watching the clock until precisely 8:59 and 59 seconds, which I figured was late enough to make a business call. I jumped into the conversation with a bit too much enthusiasm, I suppose, because my client responded with, "Whoa, you are WAY too awake for this time of morning."

I didn't tell her I'd been up for five hours and had already run two miles, answered a bunch of e-mail, studied my Bible, got four kids up, fed, dressed and off to school, done a batch of wash and weeded my herb garden. I especially didn't tell her I got up that early because I wanted to.

That hasn't always been the case. Motherhood did this to me. When my husband and I were first married, he was much more coherent in the wee hours. I'd force myself out of bed after the fifth assault of the alarm clock and relocate to the cold, hard bathroom floor desperate for a few seconds more sleep but knowing I'd be miserable enough on the floor to relent and stagger toward the shower.

Then we brought home that first little squalling bundle and my sleep habits were rearranged. We'd wanted a baby for so long that, each time I heard the glorious sound of Haley O'Hara crying for another feeding, I was determined to respond with an eager, happy face no matter how sleep deprived I was.

I never wanted her or the three babies who followed to feel that they were disturbing me or were a burden at whatever hour they decided was morning. I determined I'd be 100% Mom as soon as they called me into action.

But the real metamorphosis didn't occur until I stumbled upon a secret.

Because I was lucky enough to make raising my kids a full-time gig, our routine tended to be pretty loosey goosey. We got up when we felt like it (okay, when they felt like it) and went to bed when we were tired of being awake.

We woke up together. We went to bed together. We grocery-shopped, ran errands, ate, played and bathed together. We did everything together. Life was grand.

Then one day I realized that, if I could only make myself get up an hour before my kids, I could have sixty minutes alone in my own home—something I hadn't experienced in years.

The first day was intoxicating. I could serve myself a cup of coffee and drink it while it was still hot. I could write a letter and keep my mind on what I wanted to say. Most of my letters at that time consisted of disconnected thoughts written with two or three different pens whenever I could grab a minute, usually perched on the edge of the sandbox or sitting on the floor beside the bathtub where the kids were temporarily distracted by bubbles.

But in my stolen hour, I could read a book, exercise, listen to grown-up music and eat a leisurely breakfast. I could coax one of the cats to snuggle in my lap rather than hunker by the food bowl with one eye on whichever preschooler might decide he'd enjoy some dress-up clothes.

Even if I used my time to do laundry or wash dishes, it felt indulgent to be doing it in complete solitude. I could begin a task and see it through to completion without stopping and starting it fifteen times. I could sneak in a bath all by myself without an audience or running commentary. I bought myself grown-up bath products and adult breakfast foods—aromatherapy and English muffins, hot oil treatments and lemon curd.

I had no idea how starved I'd become for my own company and quickly honed skills that will serve me well if I ever decide to become a cat burglar. I can do anything soundlessly if it means I get to do it alone. Of course, before long, an hour wasn't enough, so I got up two hours earlier, then three and sometimes four.

More than a decade has passed since that epiphany. The kids are teenagers now and having their own morning wrangle with the snooze alarm. But I've kept my early hours to myself. I've changed my title from stay-at-home mom to work-at-home mom (from SAHM to WAHM) but that first hour or two of the morning is still my favorite time. Most days I accomplish more between 4:00 A.M. and 6:00 A.M.—when the kids wake up to sing a few bars of Mom, I need... Mom, I want... and Mom, I gotta' have... —then I do between 6:00 and bedtime.

Even though they're taller than I am, I still like the idea of my kids waking up to a pleasant mama. And after a brisk run with the dogs, some quality time with the cats, my daily Bible study, a little e-mail interaction and as much coffee as I care to drink, I'm far more chipper than my husband or kids—or my clients—would like me to be.

So that's it. That's my dirty little secret. I get up early and I like it. Besides if I ever consider a career change, I'd make one heck of a good cat burglar.

~Mimi Greenwood Knight

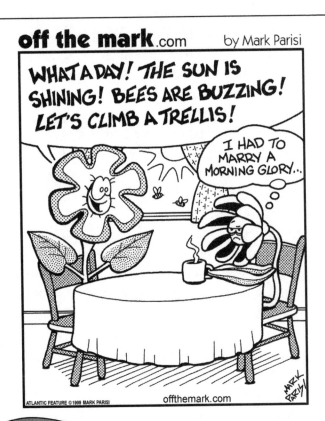

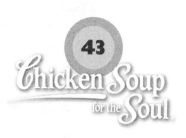

The Best Goal He Never Reached

And in the end, it's not the years in your life that count.
It's the life in your years.
~Abraham Lincoln

I love making lists. I enjoy accomplishing tasks and being able to see my progress on a sheet of paper with lines marked through it. I make shopping lists, lists for chores around the house, and projects at work. I find it incredibly motivating to put my goals on paper. And that is why, at the end of each December, I sit down at my kitchen table with paper and pen and write "The Mother List."

My New Year's list is as important to me as any other holiday tradition. Like watching the ball drop in Times Square or making a midnight champagne toast, my New Year is not official without a complete, updated list.

I make annual financial goals, career goals, fitness goals, and educational goals. Some are very realistic and are easily reached. Others are a bit more far fetched and require a lot of wishful thinking. But that's okay. January is the perfect month for high hopes and big dreams.

About seven years ago, my New Year's list included going back to school for a graduate degree. I knew it would be a difficult task for a working adult, but I had to go for it, especially once my goal was on paper. I took courses on Saturdays and Sundays and worked Monday through Friday. I was quickly reminded why I was so happy and relieved when I finally completed my undergraduate degree. The stress was overwhelming: working on papers until 3:00 A.M., sitting in class for eight hours, and dreaming about oversleeping and missing class. That actually happened only once. I finished the degree and crossed it off my list.

Four years ago, the first item on my list was to become a published writer. I had always been passionate about writing, but my credits were limited to a few high school publications and a local poetry contest. At the time, I was working for a company that published a weekly newspaper. I figured I didn't have anything to lose, so I proposed a column idea to the publisher. He liked my proposal and my first article went to press in November of that year. I reached my goal.

I wrote for that paper, the *Myrtle Beach Herald*, for a little more than two years. I wrote a column, covered a Willie Nelson and Bob Dylan concert, and interviewed numerous officials in the Myrtle Beach area and surrounding counties. But no one of political importance or celebrity status made a bigger impression on me than a lady named Rennie Lansberg.

I interviewed Mrs. Lansberg, a recent widow, for the obituary section of the paper. It was my job to find out all I could about her deceased husband and write a piece that truly captured his essence. It was the most challenging assignment I had ever been given. How do you write, in 400 words or fewer, a person's life story? How do you determine what to include and what to leave out?

Mrs. Lansberg told me that her husband, Fred, was a religious man who treasured his family and his friendships. He loved to travel, especially on all-inclusive cruise ships, and his favorite food was Philly Cheese Steak sandwiches. In fact, that was his last meal.

Fred Lansberg was the type of man anyone would be proud to call a friend. He cooked for the homeless, donated blood regularly, and worked tirelessly for his church. He was a former accountant, and though he was a dedicated employee who was named "favorite bean counter," he was equally dedicated to his social life. Fred Lansberg was often found surrounded by friends, wearing a T-shirt, shorts, flip-flops and a broad smile.

Towards the end of the emotionally draining interview, Mrs. Lansberg told me that her husband was a very goal-oriented person and that he made many lists. She said his most recent goal had been to read his father's entire collection of Charles Dickens novels. "He didn't do it though," she said. "He was too busy enjoying his life." As it turns out, it was the best goal he never reached.

The brief time I spent interviewing Rennie Lansberg has made a lasting impression on me. I think about her story often, and especially in December when I sit down to write my annual list. I have not stopped writing my list; but this experience has changed my perspective.

Last year, I accomplished most of my goals. I paid down the credit card balance, exercised more, and stopped putting sugar and cream in my coffee. But I did not get around to organizing my file cabinet, cleaning out my attic, or labeling the pictures in my digital photo album. I planned to do it but I didn't have time. I was too busy enjoying life.

~Melissa Face

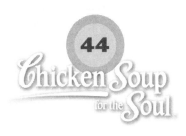

Finding a Way to Move On

I would maintain that thanks are the highest form of thought;
and that gratitude is happiness doubled by wonder.
~G.K. Chesterton

November sunlight lay in golden patches along the quiet neighborhood street. I sat on the front stoop watching a handful of leaves dance to the rhythm of an early morning breeze. We had gathered at my sister's house to celebrate Thanksgiving, but I wasn't sure I had a grateful bone in my body.

The year had been a tumultuous one. A year filled with loss and pain. In fact, I had already named it the "year of tears." From January until now, I could not recall a single day that tears had not rushed to my eyes. I wondered if the storm in my soul would ever subside. Would I spend the rest of my life struggling with this grief, nursing this awful ache in my heart?

It wasn't like me to be so wrapped up in my sorrow. I had lived through troubling times before and managed to come through with praise on my lips and a song in my heart. And even now, there had been brief periods of enjoyment, but they seemed to vanish as quickly as they came.

As I wrestled with my thoughts that autumn morning, I suddenly remembered a day when my daughter was in second grade. She came to me one afternoon and carefully handed me four small pieces of hardened clay.

"Mom," she said, looking dismal. "My world fell apart."

I didn't understand at first, but on closer inspection I could clearly see she had fashioned a world from the blue and green mixture of clay that now lay broken in my hands.

Acting like the typical fix-it-all mother, I gently led Anna into my office and, with a few pieces of tape, put her clay world back together again.

She was not impressed. "But, Mom," she said with a deep sigh. "It's got holes and cracks in it." Indeed, it did.

For years, I kept that cracked ball of clay in my desk drawer, unable to forget my child's disappointment when her "world" had fallen apart. How appropriate that I would think of it at a time like this.

Later in the afternoon, we joined hands around the table and paused for a time of prayer. With a voice soft and low, my father said, "Children, we have so much to be thankful for today."

I cannot tell you the impact that simple sentence had upon me. As my eyes swept around the table, I looked at each member of my family—all carrying burdens of their own. Yet there they sat, strong and in good health, all smiling expectantly, nodding in agreement.

It was then I realized that, at some point during my year of tears, I had simply stopped living, stuck in the rut of my pain. Something had to change.

As we bowed our heads to pray, the prayer found in the third chapter of Habakkuk became my own that day: "Though the fig tree does not bud and there are no grapes on the vines, though the olive crop fails and the fields produce no food, though there are no sheep in the pen and no cattle in the stalls, yet I will rejoice in the Lord. I will be joyful in God my Savior. The Lord God is my strength."

We returned home a few days later, and I decided to start a "blessings" journal. Though my heart remained heavy, I looked harder to find the good things in my life—things for which I was thankful—and I wrote them down.

The first few months were a struggle, not because there was nothing to record, but because my anger and grief kept surfacing. I could not see beyond the pain. I still wanted to hurt those who had wronged me.

Yet in time, this simple writing exercise changed me. I began noticing things I had often overlooked, or taken for granted. The bright red cardinal perched on the ledge outside my kitchen window went into my blessings journal. And when I stood in line at the grocery store and overheard the delightful sounds of a baby laughing, I added that to my list. The intricate shape of a leaf. The smile of a stranger at the gas station. Fresh linens on the bed. The moon's path across the water. All these simple things went into my blessings journal.

And a curious thing happened. Whenever I started counting my blessings, my heart filled up with gratitude, leaving little room for anything else.

~Dayle Allen Shockley

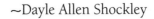

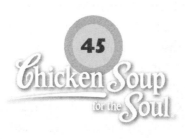

The Resolution of Silence

All men should strive
To learn before they die
What they are running from, and to, and why.
~James Thurber

When my kids were young, we'd play a game on long car trips called the "no talking game." Who could stay quiet for the longest time? None of us were very successful and quickly someone would innocently ask, "Where are the Fruit Roll-Ups?" or "Who took my shoe?" and the game was over. So when I resolved to stay quiet for ten days on a silent yoga retreat, I was apprehensive to say the least.

When I arrived at the Meditation Center, the woman at the front desk spoke softly. "Welcome and you do not have to worry about silence until later this evening." I was relieved that I would not have to use hand gestures to get oriented, as I'd never left my husband and three children, my psychotherapy practice, or my e-mail for ten days. She handed me my room key wrapped in a black cord. As I opened the door to my room, I wondered what doors would also be opened by silence.

The first evening our small group met with our yoga master. We sat on mats in a warm room with beautiful music and sipped sweet tea. Our daily schedule was printed out, each day like the next, 6:00 A.M. — morning meditation, breakfast, morning session, lunch, afternoon session, dinner, evening session, 10:00 P.M. — go to bed.

I felt like a child at a camp I wasn't sure I was going to enjoy. The evening ended with a discussion about how our daily conversations can often be distractions from honest conversations with ourselves. Quiet allows our inner voice to be heard. We were expected to be silent during the day and only speak if absolutely necessary. I wasn't sure what was defined as "absolutely necessary," so I spoke up. "Excuse me, but I usually go running every morning. Would that be possible?" "Oh no," my master answered. "What do you run from?" This was not going to be a fun camp. Silence was one thing, but I had made no running resolutions.

Our first morning meditation was before sunrise—learning to walk slowly four times around the garden pond, a little different than my four-mile run. As we nodded hello under a moonlit sky, it was a relief not to make idle conversation. We breathed slowly, white wisps of cool air. We were taught to focus on our feet—heel to toe, heel to toe. I soon learned that silently repeating "heal, soul, heal, soul" was calming. The silence spun a melody that we actually didn't want to interrupt with conversation.

Our days continued. We held yoga poses much longer than one could imagine. We did intensive exercises to strengthen ourselves, carrying us deeper into the cradle of our souls. Often all of us flew into our heads, wondering if the Caribbean might have been a better destination. But we learned true beauty lay so near, with no need for a passport. It is the small part within us that is actually huge, holding the "soul-er" power which guides us in all our life decisions.

In our silence, we tried to make sense of unhealthy patterns in our lives. My back and shoulder pain was an important metaphor. Unfortunately, I've always carried a small invisible whip—always pushing myself. I was raised in a New York suburb where we stood on tiptoes reaching for wealth, achievement and beauty. I thought about the pace of my life back home, where my husband and I worked long hours, took care of three children, a bounding puppy, and a spacious home. We prospered from having space in our home, yet felt deprived by no space in our lives. I drank in the simplicity of my retreat, filled by the emptiness of my appointment book.

Our small group shared a table in the dining hall. Always in silence, we were encouraged to eat mindfully, chewing our food thirty times before we swallowed. It wasn't easy and I often took bigger bites of tofu to be able to go the distance. We were the only silent table, and with each passing day the voices around us seemed louder and louder. Although everyone was speaking English, it sounded foreign and so fast-paced.

We could break our silence to check in with our real lives. So midweek the mother pull had me call home to hear about my daughter's new braces, and my son's report on the latest Denver Bronco victory. The frustration of cell phone reception was a gentle reminder of the challenge of bridging these two worlds. I shared with my husband my musings about a simpler life, a smaller home, a smaller caseload, yet a larger space for passion and creativity. I struggled, feeling homesick for family and my own pillow, and homesick for what lay deeper inside me as I questioned how I wanted to live my next fifty years.

It was one of the last afternoons when the gentle teacher asked, "You want to try running now?" I was both happy and scared. The challenge was "running" without "running away."

So under an Arizona blue sky I began a meditative run repeating, "heal, soul, heal, soul," as I had every morning. I learned much during that run. Remember to breathe. When you hit an uphill climb, lean into it and just keep going. Sometimes it is easier to go around a bush than to try plowing through. Don't make the journey more difficult; take the pebbles out of your shoes. Don't look too far ahead; you can lose your footing in the present. And as I jogged toward my room, I was reminded that in the end we all return to where we started. I had small blisters on my toes, which I learned was because my skin had softened in the contemplative desert air. My whole being had become more sensitive and open.

Our speaking began with our goodbyes as we all faced the challenge of bringing our quiet peace back to our red light/green light world and the loud music of our lives. We'd discovered a beautiful energy that felt like slippery soap in a morning shower—sweet smelling, but a challenge to hold.

My ten-day resolution of silence in a faraway desert was a beautiful version of the "silent game" and I returned home committed to driving my destiny versus driving myself. We decided to sell our home, and move a block away to a lovely yet simpler home. At first the children screamed and slammed doors but they have since forgiven us.

My husband and I work less and I spend more time writing. My husband finds peace as he tends his blossoming garden. I make time between patients to go to a daily yoga class. I dress more casually these days, cotton pants and light sweaters just so I don't have to change before and after class—my seams holding the quiet throughout the day. I drink more sweet tea than coffee, listen to quiet tunes that often compete with loud beats of teenage music behind bedroom doors.

Thus it is the bringing together of the East and the West, reconciling the junior prom limousine with the hybrid ways in the same family. When the children were young, evenings would get so wild, I'd scream something maternal like, "Can you guys just be quiet, so I can hear myself think!" How grateful I am that finally I was the one that took the time to stop talking long enough to hear.

~Priscilla Dann-Courtney

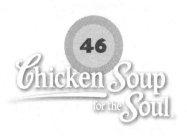

I Resolved to Make Our Own Holidays

*Every day of our lives we are on the verge of making those slight changes
that would make all the difference.*
~Mignon McLaughlin

It is a bittersweet day when we carefully wrap our holiday ornaments to store in the attic. But years ago, as I was about to take the stockings down, I thought, "If I put these away, there won't be presents in them until next December! That doesn't make sense." So I left one stocking up, where it stays all year. And every so often there's a present in it — for no reason whatsoever.

Sometimes my husband Bob or I will say to each other, "Have you checked the stocking?" It's never anything big — maybe a candy bar or a crossword puzzle book.

Every Christmas, we have an elegant dinner by candlelight. This year, as I felt glowingly aware of the uniqueness of the day, time stopped for me in a moment of bliss. And I said to Bob, "Why can't more days be like this?"

"They can't," he said. "This day is special because it comes once a year."

"But that's just in our minds. Life's too short to limit celebrations to what it says on a calendar."

We were savoring Yorkshire pudding when Bob said, "If we had this more often, we wouldn't appreciate it."

"Who says? Every summer when you bite into a lusciously ripe home-grown tomato, you close your eyes in a state of nirvana. Would you want one tomato a year?"

"No," he laughed. "But holidays are different."

"I think you're wrong. It's all what we tell ourselves. I don't want to wait until next December to feel holiday joy."

"But that's when the season comes."

"Why hold off until a certain date to rejoice?" I said. "We don't need an excuse to celebrate. Can't we resolve to make our own tradition of, let's say... having the first day of each month a make-your-own holiday? It doesn't have to be a huge deal. And it's only twelve days a year. We could do something special, like order take-out Chinese food—and eat it by candlelight."

On Christmas, Bob gave me a beautiful glass snow globe. When I gently shake it, snowflakes softly whirl around a dainty evergreen tree. On each limb is a tiny red candle. It's magical to watch the snow swirl as it slowly settles around the tree. And it brings back memories. When I was a little girl I'd watch snow twirl around a ballerina in a globe, making her seem alive as the flakes made their way toward her pink ballet slippers.

I'm not putting Bob's gift away, even though it's a Christmas scene. It's too beautiful to store in the attic. So it will rest on my mantle where I can treasure its beauty. And my favorite ornament, a hand painted oyster shell from Cape Cod, and of course the stocking, will stay downstairs so we can savor more bliss all year long.

I don't want to miss any potential for festivity. Why would I? Where is it written that corned beef is only for St. Patrick's Day or maple-glazed ham for Easter? Plus, must we wait for friends' birthdays to give them presents?

And so, we both made the resolution to celebrate the first day of every month. "If we don't set the date, we may not do it," I said.

And frankly, I think making our own traditions is just as meaningful as conventional rituals. Because they don't come from a calendar. They come from the love in one's heart.

~Saralee Perel

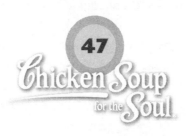

Simpler Resolutions

Be content with what you have, rejoice in the way things are.
When you realize there is nothing lacking, the whole world belongs to you.
~Lao Tzu

I have always kept my New Year's resolutions in a file. They're fun to look back on, to chart my accomplishments or to see where I need to work harder.

But looking back at my resolutions from two years ago, I barely recognize my goals against the backdrop of the life I live now.

Two years ago, I aimed for a weight loss of ten to fifteen pounds and promised myself laser treatment for the bags under my eyes.

I vowed to travel more with my husband and to take a vacation or two with my mom, as I'd done in years past. I planned to visit a dear friend I hadn't seen in a couple of years. Work was also high on my list. More writing was to be done and I was going to sell a book idea I'd had for a long time. At the end of my list was a brief mention about keeping my family, people and animals alike, healthy.

Little did I know the complete upheaval that lay ahead for me.

The first few months of the New Year went along as planned. Then in May, my ninety-three-year-old mother fell, fracturing a hip and wrist. At her delicate age, the fear was not just how she'd heal from the required surgery, but would she even survive it at all? She spent the next month in the hospital and rehab, while I spent each day at her bedside. When she went home, I stayed with her day and night, putting my husband and our two dogs on the back burner. Phone calls had to suffice for the time being.

Eventually, caregivers were found and a semi-normal routine was reached where I spent part of my time with Mom and part of my time at home.

Without warning a few months later, my husband Kenny ended up in the hospital with blood pressure issues.

Soon after, one of our beloved dogs, David, was diagnosed with cancer. Since his age, too, is advanced, we feared he might not survive the surgery, let alone come through it tumor-free and healthy once again.

Those ten to fifteen pounds I wanted to lose? I still have them. The puffiness under my eyes that laser treatment was going to erase? Still there.

And travel: Does to and from vets, the hospital, doctors and grocery stores count?

My writing career? For a long time I was too tired to read, let alone write anything. And yet, I've come to see that there's a plan here. My appearance is less critical to me now. I'm looking in the mirror less because I have less time to do so. I'd rather be talking to my husband during the time we have together, or hugging our two dogs.

My satisfaction comes when the vet says David remains cancer-free. When I call my mom and she sounds stronger than the day before, my heart leaps.

Instead of resenting the turn my life has taken, I'm trying to appreciate the new experiences it has brought. From her chair, my mom has taught me how to make the cinnamon rolls she always made for me when I was a child.

She's re-introduced me to the fun of sewing as she supervises my completion of projects she'd begun before her fall.

I've realized that I've relieved Mom of some of the household responsibilities she so strongly performed for ninety-three years. She deserves it!

In the process of taking part-time care of her cat I've found another pet to love—one that I used to just greet casually when I visited.

My writing career is now up and running again. I've found new locations to write that I never tried before—doctor's waiting rooms, a quiet moment before breakfast, while waiting for dinner to finish cooking.

Each night before I go to sleep, I say thank you for the gift of life we've all been given for another day. It's not a perfect life for any of us. It's not glamorous or worldly. But it's filled with what I now count as truly important things: love and health, small triumphs and simple joys.

My resolutions will reflect that from now on. And if I can accomplish those few, precious things, life will be complete.

~Valerie Porter

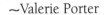

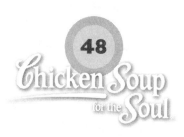

Check the Cart

Beware of little expenses;
a small leak will sink a great ship.
~Benjamin Franklin

As a single mom working several jobs, I accounted for every penny. My son's needs came first, then the rent and groceries, then the rest of the bills. Every month, I intended to save for that proverbial rainy day, but it just didn't happen. As frugal as I tried to be, the expense column topped out the income on my monthly budget.

Then one day, I discovered a game I could play to find those extra pennies. I called it my Cart Check game.

Every time I shopped at the big box stores and then rolled my cart toward the check-out line, I looked through my items. Was there something I could do without? That filigreed T-shirt that I was certain would look great with a denim skirt? It was only $4—a real bargain—but couldn't I do without it? I took it back to the misses section and congratulated myself on saving $4.

The same strategy worked for groceries. Although I followed my list and used coupons, invariably a hunger pang would strike and I would end up with something extra. So I played the Cart Check game. Rolling toward the check-out, I looked through the cart. That package of cookies might be my son's favorites, but did he really need the extra sugar? Put it back and save $2.98.

As my son grew, we played the game together. Go up and down

the aisles and select what we need. Then roll to the check-out and do the Cart Check. My shampoo bottle wasn't completely empty yet. I could wait another week, dilute it further with water, and maybe find a coupon when it was completely gone. A savings of $3.95.

My son looked through the cart, "Here, Mom. We don't need this toothpaste."

"Yes, we do. Every night we brush our teeth. But how about these toy cars? What if we buy only one instead of two?"

"Well, okay."

I rewarded Chad by giving him the 88 cents we had saved.

Our Cart Check game helped us save each time we shopped and kept us from impulse spending. Gradually, we made it through those hard times, and I raised Chad to consider the importance of saving. We're both still careful about shopping, and we still use the Cart Check game whenever he visits me and we shop together.

Now that the economy is in a critical state and every penny counts, I'm making a resolution to re-install Cart Check into my weekly shopping. It's too easy to add an extra lipstick or a new towel to my shopping list, not realizing how much those impulsive choices add to my monthly bills. But this time, I plan to introduce a twist in the game.

After my Cart Check, I'll add up the amount I've saved and put that money in a special account. By the end of the year, I should have a nice sum that I can use for Christmas gifts. Or maybe I'll give it to another single mom who's struggling with expenses.

The Cart Check game will then not only help me and leave a legacy for my son, but also help another mother balance her budget and make it to the end of the month.

~Rebecca Jay

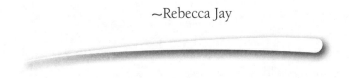

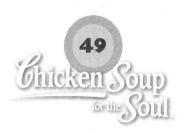

One House, Two Faces

Life is really simple, but we insist on making it complicated.
~Confucius

My first house was so small the living room did triple duty as a library, office and dining room. Although I had an eat-in kitchen, I ate most of my meals in my favorite black leather chair, surrounded by my books.

As a result, my living room always had what I called a lived-in look and what my mother called a mess. Books, file folders, and newspapers littered the floor. Empty glasses and plates often lay scattered across the coffee table. And cat toys hid between the couch cushions waiting for unwary visitors.

When visitors were due, I went into hyper-drive. I dusted, vacuumed and lugged all the books and papers upstairs where I hid them in my bedroom behind closed doors. By the time my guests arrived, the living room looked showroom perfect.

I, on the other hand, often felt frazzled and couldn't enjoy my guests. Sometimes I resented them, as if they were forcing my house and me to be something we weren't—to put on our company face, rather than our real face.

One house, two faces.

After they left, the living room soon returned to its usual cluttered look and I could relax again.

After eight years, I decided it was time for a change. Figuring that bigger was better, I moved up in size for my next house, adding about a third more square footage. Not only did I have a full office, but I also had a den off my kitchen, the main reason I bought the house. I did all my reading and most of my eating there, as well as watching TV.

My combined living and dining room, which took up half of the first floor, were like the old time parlors—unused except for company. The only things missing were a rope strung across the entrance and an "Off Limits" sign.

While the front of the house remained neat and company-ready, and mostly unused, those rooms had a sterile look and feel to them. No books piled on the coffee table. No cat toys strung across the floor. No cushions thrown haphazardly on the couch.

The back of the house, where the real "living" went on, had the warmth and lived-in look that was lacking in the formal rooms; yet guests seldom saw that part of the house.

Some days, I felt as if I were living in a house with two faces: One reserved for company and the other for me.

Over the next six years, a sense of dissatisfaction seeped into the house and into me. Each year I watched my utility bills and taxes rise, taking a bigger and bigger chunk of my salary. A sobering session with my calculator showed me I was now working one full month a year just to pay the overhead for that extra space.

I was locked into a job I no longer liked for the sake of a grander house. My dream home had turned into an albatross.

I had two choices: Start charging my guests an admission fee or sell the house. Since my house wasn't on a par with the stately homes of Britain, I chose option #2.

By the end of that year. I made two changes. I sold my house and moved into a considerably smaller one. And I used the difference in house prices to buy myself two years of freedom to explore new job possibilities.

It's been seven years since I moved. I'm back to a tiny office and once more living in my "living" room. And I love it.

Now when guests are invited over, I do a little tidying up instead of a whirlwind mega-cleaning. I pile the books a bit more neatly and clear a space on the coffee table for tea and cake. As my guests arrive, they're met by a relaxed hostess who has the energy to enjoy her company and a cluttered, lived-in room that shouts, "Real people really live here."

You know something? None of my guests has ever complained. In fact, they generally comment on how homey the house feels.

My house is no longer two-faced. The face it shows guests is the same one it shows me. And if that face is a little wrinkled and time-worn, well, so is mine.

~Harriet Cooper

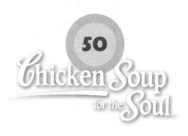

50

Resolving to Honor Memories

Leftovers in their less visible form are called memories.
Stored in the refrigerator of the mind and the cupboard of the heart.
~Thomas Fuller

The first time I walked into my mother's apartment after she died, I turned and bolted. The smell of her perfume, the sight of her eyeglasses, her magazines, her comb—and the absence of her—were just too much.

I couldn't go back for days.

But no matter how much I wanted to avoid it, there was the inevitable sad work of clearing out the place where Mom had lived for thirty-seven years. And nobody can prepare you for going through the personal effects of a parent you've loved and lost. If grief is an ambush, this sorting out is its handmaiden.

Ultimately, I took huge cartons, and with my husband's help, stockpiled the things I couldn't bear to part with. There was no rhyme or reason to this process—just pure instinct.

How could I leave behind the shoebox filled to the brim with every card we'd ever sent her, ordinary cards I'd picked out in a moment without even deliberating over the message? Every sappy birthday card and Mother's Day card was there, dated, and in its original envelope. Why hadn't I sent her nicer ones?

No matter where I went in the apartment there was something destined to stop me in my tracks and make me sob.

But I pushed on.

I scooped up the predictable things—my mother's china, the paintings that had been in my life since childhood, because they were part of the landscape of our house, and the scarves that still carried her scent.

Those cartons came back to our house, with my husband showing remarkable and loving patience with the excesses. And they got stashed in the basement, where I wouldn't see them often, let alone open them.

And that might have been that.

Except that one day during the spring after Mom's death, I had a reckoning: I was entertaining, and knew that a beautiful English casserole that my mother had loved would make a perfect centerpiece for our table, especially if I filled it with her recipe for Swedish meatballs.

That day, I made a promise to myself, one I wasn't at all sure I could keep: I would stop avoiding the bits and pieces of Mom's life—the tangible evidence of her world in the apartment that had claimed and framed her days. Gradually, I would integrate them into my life.

I would begin with that casserole dish, one of her prized possessions, and her recipe box that contained the careful directions for her famous Swedish meatballs.

I would love to say that I simply did it. That I kept my resolve strong. But it took me a full week to bring myself just to open the first carton and pull out that lovely oval dish. Touching it made me weep.

It was somehow easier to dig out the recipe, and to place Mom's old wooden recipe box in a kitchen cabinet, out of sight for now, but not out of mind.

Small things marked enormous progress: I now carry my mother's deep blue eyeglass case in my own pocketbook. Initially, just seeing it among my things stunned me. But then I began to love its familiarity: how many times had I seen my dear mother reach for that case? She had loved it. Now I love it, too.

My mother's pearls are often around my neck. It took a while until that stopped feeling weird. Now it feels wonderful.

On cold days, I wear my mother's blue flannel bathrobe, the one I pulled out of the Goodwill pile at the last minute. "As old as the hills," my mother used to say, "but it's warm." That was enough of a rave for me.

But perhaps nothing is woven into my days and nights as completely and joyfully as the most unexpected of items.

One Mother's Day, late in Mom's life, we gifted her with a set of red cookware—spunky and modern. At first, she insisted that we take it all back. Finally, she agreed to keep just one piece: a little red pot.

No utensil was ever more lovingly cared for. Mom polished it to a gleam, delighted to see something bright and new in what had become a weary kitchen.

That pot now sits on my stove. I use it as often as I can, and cherish it, because she did.

My resolution to keep my mother "with me" may sound foolish, even macabre.

But that little red pot stands as a symbol of what has turned out to be one of the most important resolutions of my life: to honor my mother by surrounding myself with the things she wore and touched and used.

I've learned through this resolve that there's great comfort in the mundane.

And that a little red pot can make remembering an act of love.

~Sally Friedman

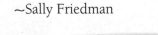

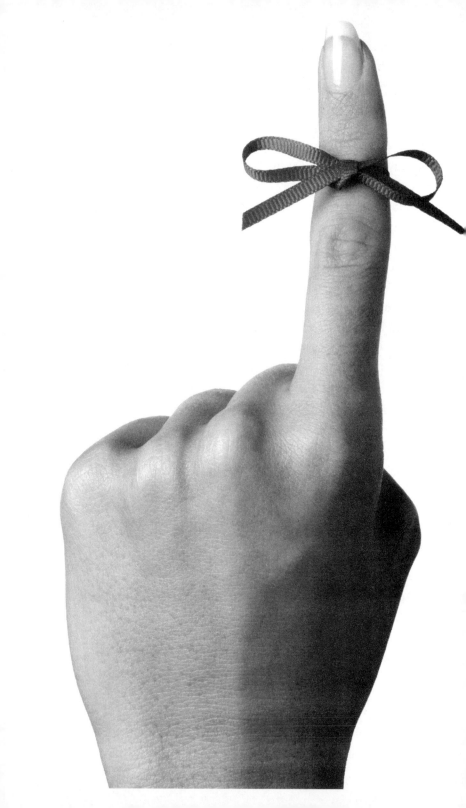

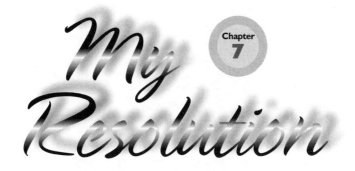

Chapter 7

My Resolution

I Did It!

Shoot for the moon. Even if you miss, you'll land among the stars.

~Les Brown

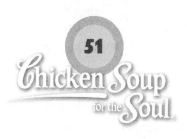

Churchill and Me

Say "Yes" to the seedlings and a giant forest cleaves the sky.
Say "Yes" to the universe and the planets become your neighbors.
Say "Yes" to dreams of love and freedom.
It is the password to utopia.
~Brooks Atkinson

After twenty-nine years as editor of a travel magazine, when I turned seventy-eight, I was persuaded to retire and give someone younger an opportunity to continue the publication. I had my little toy poodle Nikolas as a companion. I had my pension fund and my 401K... enough to live on comfortably. I had a condo on the beach. My three children were spread across the world... England, Denver, Washington. They and their children were all doing well. What more could I want?

I had had a hip replacement in 2001. Now, at eighty, my knee was wearing out, and I was contemplating another slow and painful joint replacement. All three children were urging me to come live with them, and I was grateful for their loving concern, but somehow that was a signal that my life was over, my independence was gone. What did I really have to live for? My depression was all consuming.

One morning, when I was at my lowest ebb, I read one of those self-help columns in the daily newspaper. What caught my eye was the lead line: Confidential "Should I Continue or Quit?" The adviser wrote the following: The answer to your question will be found in this profound statement that originated with Sir Winston Churchill.

"To each there comes in their lifetime a special moment when they are figuratively tapped on the shoulder and offered the chance to do a very special thing, unique to them and fitted to their talents. What a tragedy if that moment finds them unprepared or unqualified for that which could have been their finest hour."

I sat bolt upright in my chair. That message was aimed directly at me. What was this special thing, unique to me and fitted to my talents? Editing a magazine. But who was going to hire an eighty-year-old woman? What a preposterous idea! I threw away the newspaper and felt myself slipping back into my depression. But what did Churchill say? "What a tragedy if that moment finds them unprepared?" I certainly was qualified. What was it my mother used to say to me? "Find a need and fill it."

I drove to the grocery store and looked at the hundreds of magazines on the racks... sports magazines, travel magazines, home decorating magazines... every subject under the sun. What could possibly be the need there? Ah, but they were all national magazines.

What was specifically designed for condos on the beach? We shared the same problems... beach nourishment, threatened hurricanes, rising taxes and lowering property values.

Who was addressing those particular questions, and on the lighter side, who was telling residents where to dine locally, where to shop, what to see and do in the area?

My mind began to race. What if I started my own magazine? What if I addressed the concerns and interests of condo residents on the beach? It didn't have to be a national magazine... it could be totally local, supported by local advertisers. There were twenty condo complexes on my barrier island. What if I just printed a quarterly publication that would go to 5,000 readers?

I began to kick around names. As each new title came to me, I'd check the Internet to see if it was available. Great idea... oh, someone already thought of that. After testing dozens of names, the perfect one came to me. It was for beach residents... it had to have "Beach" in the title. And it had to be interactive with beach residents... Beach Thoughts... Beach Notes... *Beach Talk*! Incredibly, *Beach Talk* was not registered. I signed up for a domain immediately and registered the name.

It was January, 2007. I resolved I would take $5,000 from my savings account to cover start-up costs and launch *Beach Talk Magazine* within six months.

I called the printer with whom I had done business for twenty years. Together we had built a travel magazine from 200,000 circulation to 4.5 million. Could he help me? Sadly, his company wouldn't consider printing less than 30,000 magazines, and I was thinking in the neighborhood of 5,000 tops to get started. Why did I think it would be easy?

I turned to the phone book, and after a dozen calls, I found a local web offset printer who agreed that he would print a four-color 40-page magazine on 50 lb. stock for what I considered was a reasonable price. I was off and running.

A major cost would be postage. At $1.31 per magazine, I'd go through my $5,000 before I even paid the printer. What if I delivered the magazines to each condo myself? How many boxes could my three-year-old Cadillac carry without tearing out the transmission? If I made two trips—it could be done. I resolved to do it myself.

What about writers? A handful of writers from my previous travel magazine were eager to help me get started. The rest of the articles I'd write myself and put relatives' names as bylines. The majority of the photos I took with a little digital camera.

I enlisted the support of each condominium by taking a photo of the condo manager and writing an accompanying profile. They were more than willing to accept delivery of the magazine every three months.

Then I compiled articles about the beach. "Shell Game"... how to make a sea shell lamp. "Diary of a Beach Wedding"... a resident's niece was married on the beach. "Let's Talk Sailing"... a story about local sailing lessons. In no time I had gathered or written enough articles, with photos, to fill forty pages.

With a mock-up in hand, I called on local restaurants and shops and managed to sell enough ads to cover the first printing bill.

By June 1, 2007, I was delivering the Premiere Edition of *Beach Talk Magazine*.

And this week, a new knee in place, in the same sagging Cadillac, I delivered the June 2008 issue of *Beach Talk Magazine* exactly one year and five issues later.

Depression? I don't have time for that. My resolution has been fulfilled. As Winston Churchill had said, "What a tragedy if that moment had found me unprepared."

~Phyllis W. Zeno

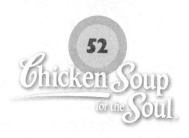

52

Tarnished Hero

The kindest word in all the world is the unkind word, unsaid.
~Author Unknown

At a recent high school reunion, I saw Colin again. After forty-five years, his looks have changed quite a bit. He has white hair now rather than dark curls. He didn't recognize me, but knowing I was a high school classmate from bygone days, he hugged me like an old friend. Time has mellowed him.

He is, in a sense, my tarnished hero.

I'll explain.

In that long ago fourteenth year, my mirror revealed exactly what I wanted to see of myself. It ignored the bath scale recording my weight creeping up, up, up. My bedroom full-length mirror played denial right along with me, convincing me that I'd not changed a lick, and was, in fact, quite normal.

My family, too, practiced see-no-evil. Observing me day in, day out, they did not, for a long time, detect my bulging shape beneath big shirts and baggy jeans.

One day in homeroom, my teacher sent me to deliver some papers to the principal's office. As I left the class, Colin, quite the artist, began to garnish the door with spring decorations. I shyly excused myself to pass and he politely stepped aside, then closed the door behind me.

In eighth grade, Colin was—if not the most verbose and friendly—quite handsome and popular with the girls. I, too, was secretly smitten. My romantic mind painted him dark and mysterious, with ebony eyes that, on occasion, flicked over me with maddening unreadableness.

The principal's office was in another building and I enjoyed the warm sunshine as I strolled across campus and back. When I approached the door to my classroom, I spied Colin through the high, small window, tongue poked between perfect teeth, his good-looking face tense with concentration as he continued to arrange his handiwork on the door. The other classmates worked and chatted away during this free morning time.

I paused to pat down my hair, took a deep breath and gently turned the knob, a tentative motion so as not to abruptly interrupt Colin's creativity. He stepped back, a moment I used to crack the door open and step across the threshold, intending to move past him and allow him to resume his artwork.

I gazed up at him, forming an apologetic smile. It was then that I saw his black eyes turn stormy. "Hurry up, Fatso," he muttered through his teeth, in a voice low and unfeeling.

Shock melted my smile as he stood there, tall and imperial, his impatience and disdain snapping at me like an enraged Rottweiler. Now I knew what thoughts lay behind those mystical eyes.

For one long instant, hurt and humiliation opted to curl me into a fetal knot right there at his feet. But in the next heartbeat, anger stirred deep, deep inside me and I met his gaze defiantly, seeing him for the first time, seeing past his male beauty into an insensitive soul, one that greatly diminished him.

I flounced past him and took my seat, fighting back tears. Thank God nobody else had heard his callous words. I glimpsed his reflection in the glass where he worked, nonchalant and softly whistling.

Why, he doesn't even care that he's hurt me.

My umbrage grew and burgeoned in the next twenty-four hours, hours during which I gazed in my mirror and saw, really saw the blobs of fat that buried my bone structure and caricaturized me. Didn't my family see my chipmunk cheeks? Why hadn't anybody told me?

Somebody did. I clamped my teeth together.

Colin did.

"Never again," I vowed, "would I be the target of such ridicule."

My resolution was cemented firmly into place and I commenced plotting. I wrote to Dr. George Crane, a medical doctor newspaper columnist and the next week received his famous *Lose Ten Pounds In Ten Days Diet* in my self-addressed stamped envelope. The diet's initial quick loss was intended only as a successful launch that would help keep one on the 900 calories (the pound a day starting point) and gradually migrate to 1,400 calories (slower loss), which I maintained for the long haul.

"Oh yes, Colin," I muttered through my teeth daily, "I'll show YOU!"

Summer vacation began and so did my regimen. My calorie count rarely exceeded 1,200, even when my flesh screamed for more. Not even when my dad, scowling at how my shirts and jeans hung like tents on me, shoved food under my nose, heaped more mashed potatoes and gravy on my plate, and snarled, "Eat!"

I learned the art of pushing food around on my dish until it appeared nearly gone.

If my resolve threatened to waver, a flash of Colin's arrogant sneer and his "Hurry up, Fatso" snapped it firmly back into place.

By mid-summer, I'd shrunk out of my old clothes. Mom took me shopping for a new church dress—I still wore the old jeans and big shirts at home most of the time. After dressing for church that week, I spied myself in the mirror. Why, I actually had a waistline. When I walked through the den, Daddy's mouth fell open.

"Susie Q—you've really lost weight, haven't you?" I heard the worry in his voice. In Dad's family, where most of the females are "solid," my encroaching thinness, to him, equated frailty.

"Yup." I almost giggled at his astonishment. Maybe soon, he'd adjust to my new image and appreciate all my efforts. In the meantime, I'd simply keep on trucking under my own steam. I was only halfway to my goal.

The following weeks passed swiftly as I served myself small portions, eating green beans instead of rice and gravy, sliced tomatoes rather than macaroni pie, and opting for an extra piece of skinless white chicken in lieu of chocolate cake. I learned to enjoy a single homemade biscuit rather than eating three or four. I mastered juggling calories to cover small portions of treats I loved, therefore avoiding a sense of deprivation. Some weeks I lost less than others, so I stopped weighing myself as often to avoid disappointment.

Suddenly, September was upon me. Mom and I shopped for my school wardrobe. Lo and behold, I was a size eight. Standing five-feet-four, at 115 pounds, I'd reached my goal. My weight loss totaled 35 pounds.

Other things had changed during the summer. My diet had given me a clear, smooth complexion. My hair, once oily, now sported a healthy gloss. Mom took me for a fashionable haircut. The different "do" becomingly hugged my newly oval face, completing my metamorphosis.

What satisfaction I experienced by sticking to my resolution. Little did I know that it equipped me with lifelong self-confidence and propelled me into being an above-average achiever.

The first day back at school, I was a mite bewildered when many of my friends walked past without acknowledging me. Finally, I took the initiative to approach them and was astonished that they didn't know me! Without fail, this wild look of disbelief washed over their features as recognition dawned. I felt gratified, seeing they were excited that I'd reached out and taken charge of my destiny.

I looked for him. Colin. The old anger still stirred when I recalled his insult; but not as forcefully. Still—I wanted to confront him, to see his reaction. At the end of the day, I'd still not spotted him.

"Where's Colin?" I finally asked his old buddy, George.

"Oh, Colin's moved to Conastee," replied George, his puzzled, appreciative gaze roaming my face. "Uh—who are you?"

"Susie Miller."

"No! It can't be!"

I strolled away, a bit disappointed that Colin wouldn't see the new me.

Then, quite suddenly, it ceased to matter. Because I now had a life and in the days that followed, I grew to realize that the guys' little asides to me were not taunts but flirts. I slowly accepted the fact that I was attractive and well liked by my peers.

My self-confidence snapped into place.

Soon, I began to see Colin simply as the unknowing catalyst that had propelled me from there to here, who had forced me to see me for who I was—an out of control, overeating person. He sparked the anger that fueled my purpose, one that rescued me from smothering beneath masses of fat and cellulite, from a life of loneliness and heartbreak. He crash-landed me into vanity—not the evil kind—the healthy, survival, feel good kind.

Seeing Colin again, forty-five years later, at the high school reunion gave me closure. Seeing his own paunch and imperfections helped me to forgive him for his adolescent insensitivity. He's not the same after all this time. Wisdom, somewhere along the way, caught up with him. I never told him about that time because I'm certain he would be horrified and repentant. It no longer matters. We've remained friends in recent years, we and our spouses seeing each other on a regular basis, loving and respecting each other.

I surprise even myself by seeing him as a different kind of hero, one not spawned from nobility. Or kindness... one even ignorant of his hero-status. A hero, nevertheless, because I can't help but ask myself at times, "Had it not been for the Colin episode, would I have ever faced up to my problem and made my first adult resolution?"

Who knows? All I know is that every time the scale needle begins to creep up, I need only to hear yesteryear's "Hurry up, Fatso," to revive my resolve.

And I tighten my lips, square my shoulders, and quietly renew my resolution, "Never again."

Thanks, Colin.

~Emily Sue Harvey

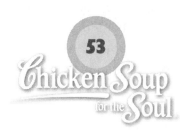

53

I Shot the Sheriff

A good snapshot stops a moment from running away.
~Eudora Welty

I admit it—I shot the traffic cop, but I had a good reason. After I made the illegal right turn, his motorcycle zoomed into my rearview mirror. Dang! I pulled to the curb and meekly handed over my license and registration. He strolled behind the car. Turning, I regarded him through the back window as he wrote the citation. His helmet gleamed in the sunlight, white against the red and yellow leaves of the liquidambar trees. I reached into my bag, my hand closing around the comforting, shiny black object I was never without. Raising it above the seat, I fixed the helmet in my sights. With a steady hand, I snapped the shutter.

I was fulfilling my 2004 New Year's resolution; to take at least one photo each day. I'd made it this far, and I wasn't going to abandon the project. The police officer was my photo for November 3rd.

I'd made the resolution on New Year's Eve. My new digital camera was still in the box because I was resistant to learning its baffling terminology—JPEG, CCD, TTL, TIFF. Yet I knew I needed to join the Digital Age. I resolved to create a visual record of the coming year. How hard could it be to grab a snapshot each day?

I began carrying my camera everywhere, looking for beautiful or intriguing subjects. Each evening I downloaded that day's photos and designated one as the official "Photo of the Day." I subscribed to a photo-sharing website and posted my daily images—landscapes, still lifes, abstracts—to my home page.

After a few weeks, I told family and friends about my resolution. They thought it was a little weird, but most of them posed willingly or didn't get too mad if I caught them in a candid moment. I snapped photos of my friend Jean with her new Honda Element one day, operating her printing press another day. I captured my husband several times—hiking, grilling steaks or reading the paper.

At first I was reluctant to approach strangers. No, make that terrified. But I wanted my collection to document the community as well as my own activities. One day in January, picketers were marching in front of the supermarket. When I grabbed the camera, it almost slid from my sweaty palms. I asked two workers to pose with their signs so that I could post their photo on my website. They exchanged an is-she-loony? look. My "Photo of the Day" explanation sounded lame even to me. Then one man said, "Okay, we're doing this to get our message across. Fire away."

It got easier each time. I took a picture of a Nordstrom saleswoman, a clerk at the Italian market, a knife-twirling chef at a Japanese restaurant. After a few months I started getting bossy: "Hold your saxophone like this," I said to the jazz player, "and turn to the left." But people didn't seem to mind, because I tried to learn something about each one. The man in the botanical garden who was polishing a bench's brass plaque said it was a memorial to his recently-deceased wife. The handsome couple running a Greek food stand at the Los Angeles County Fair told me they'd given up high-powered careers in order to pursue their dream of a nomadic life selling gyros and spanikopita.

Not everyone cooperated. One day at the dry cleaner's, I asked the proprietress to pose by the moving clothes rack for a portrait. "Oh, no!" she said, blushing. "Hair not good today!" I switched off the camera.

Another time I was zooming in on a blueberry tart at the bakery (the gum-chewing clerk had shrugged an "okay" when I'd asked permission) when the baker stormed out of the kitchen, toque aquiver and bushy eyebrows drawn together. "What are you doing?" he thundered. "We serve a unique product here!" I assured him I was not a spy from a rival bakery, but tucked my camera away nevertheless.

It was the only New Year's resolution I ever kept. At the end of 2004, I had 366 photos on my website and printed in a book—an indelible record of the year, and hard evidence that each day of our lives is unique. Photos of the Rosetta Stone in the British Museum and the towering monoliths of Stonehenge remind me of a trip to England. My nephew playing his senior percussion recital at Juilliard, a picnic overlooking the Grand Canyon, a smog-free day in downtown Los Angeles—I'd probably remember those events even without the photos.

It's the quiet domestic scenes I would have forgotten—a kettle of French onion soup simmering on the stove, the redbud tree in bloom, a scattering of golden apricot leaves lying on a weathered bench. These photos, so mundane when I took them, have gained in value. They glow with a patina of nostalgia.

I have proof that nothing lasts. The orange grove where I picnicked with friends has since been plowed under for a housing development; the rusty motel sign on an Arizona back road was torn down soon after.

And family members look different today than they did arrayed on the front porch on Thanksgiving of 2004. The little boy coloring a starfish in one photo now wields a baseball bat instead of a purple crayon. The doll being clutched so lovingly by a little girl in another photo now sits neglected on a shelf. Life changes in such tiny twitches, you don't even notice them.

By the end of the year, my camera had become an extension of my arm. I could change white balance, turn off the pop-up flash and increase ISO without even looking. I changed too. Over the course of twelve months I gradually became family archivist, photojournalist, fine art photographer and portrait artist. And cop "shooter." I never imagined I would do such a thing, but when you're desperate for a "Photo of the Day," you take any opportunity life hands you.

~Kathryn Wilkens

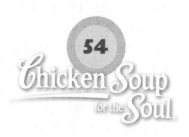

Moose O' My Heart

Goals are dreams with deadlines.
~Diana Scharf Hunt

The year was quickly slipping by when I received a phone call reminding me of my New Year's resolution.

"Hey, Mom!" greeted Elizabeth, my daughter. "It's October and you haven't fulfilled your promise to yourself."

Ah yes, my goal: to see a real, live moose by the end of the year, which seemed near impossible given that I live in the San Francisco Bay Area.

Elizabeth, ever resourceful, offered another idea.

"Catch a plane up here and we'll drive to Yellowstone for a couple of days of moose hunting," she suggested.

Montana, now that seemed possible.

"Okay," I blurted out before thinking. "I'll do it."

And I did.

Two weeks later, I was winging my way to Bozeman, where Elizabeth was a graduate student in the Science and Natural History Documentary Filmmaking Program at Montana State University. She filmed in Yellowstone quite frequently and had reported seeing moose strolling by on numerous occasions.

Moose—majestic, magical and a little ornery by most accounts. The long-legged creatures have enchanted me for as long as memory serves. Baby moose are the only mammals born with their eyes wide open, which delights me. A bowl of moose stew allows you to travel twice as fast, which intrigues me.

The two-hour drive from Bozeman to the North Entrance of Yellowstone was filled with coffee, donuts and girl talk. As we entered the Roosevelt Arch, possibility filled the air. Somewhere—everywhere—within the vast 2.2 million-acre park, moose roamed.

As do buffalo, I soon discovered. If my New Year's resolution had been to see a real, live buffalo, I would have been in heaven. Within the first ten minutes of driving into the park, herds of buffalo appeared to the left, to the right, and in the middle of the road.

The next several hours brought visions of mule deer, coyotes, and hoards of elk herds. We hiked the Fountain Paint Pot Nature Trail, photographed Mammoth Hot Springs and toured the museum at the Norris Geyser Basin. Lunchtime found us picnicking in the fall-like sunshine in the Upper Geyser Basin, recording every second until Old Faithful gave us a show. While we couldn't have asked for a more exhilarating time, we both acknowledged the absence of moose.

Disappointment loomed.

While studying a map of the park, Elizabeth recalled an area where moose had crossed her path on a previous trip. Foot to the metal, we landed at the trailhead of the Biscuit Basin. She parked the car, and I immediately got out and walked over to a ravine to peer out.

Nothing.

Since we were visiting during off-season, we had passed a total of four cars throughout the trip. But at that moment, a car pulled up alongside ours. A woman slid out from the driver's seat, and glanced my way.

"Are you looking for moose?" she yelled.

"Yes!" I yelled back.

"We just saw one—half mile down the road—left-hand side—in the bog," she directed.

"Thanks!" I yelped.

How did she know? Did my slow, apprehensive gait give me

away? Did my face mirror my sagging hopes? Did my body language convey disappointment? Perhaps my navy blue sweater bearing a big, white moose on the front gave her a clue.

Foot to the metal once again, Elizabeth sped south as four piercing eyes focused on the odometer. At exactly a half mile, Elizabeth stopped the car and we both jumped out—my daughter with her beloved camera; me with hope in my heart.

Elizabeth spotted her first. A cow moose nestled on the shore of the bog, sunbathing blissfully in the afternoon warmth.

"There she is!" she announced proudly.

A moose! A real, live moose!

We, the three of us, spent the next two hours together. Elizabeth snapping photos at an alarming rate; Ms. Moose peering at us cautiously, but trusting our intentions; and me, basking in the glow of a New Year's resolution fulfilled.

It is said that God gives us certain moments so that we may have roses in December.

Yellowstone. A spectacular October afternoon. My two girls and me.

Roses, without a doubt.

~Patricia Smith

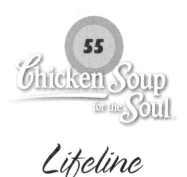

55

Lifeline

What is possible? What you will.
~Augustus William Hare

I almost overlooked the newspaper article that morning. Pain and depression from Fibromyalgia were having a field day, sapping my energy and concentration. My good days were dwindling. Depression keened after my Mom's heart bypass surgery. Four weeks later, she remained in ICU, near comatose.

It seemed unbearable at times, seeing her suffer.

It was on that morose note that I spotted the news story. "Hey, Lee," I called to my husband from the kitchen table. "Look at this. Senior citizens can go to University of South Carolina Upstate tuition-free." I shook my head. "There's got to be a catch here somewhere."

He read it over my shoulder. "Check it out."

More curious than anything, I did just that. A phone call reassured me that I had gotten it right. I could register within the week and begin January classes.

Reality set in. Dear Lord, how am I going to go to school when I can hardly drag myself out of bed some days?

Yet stopping just a few credit hours short of my English degree was one of the deep regrets of my life. Years earlier, changes in location, occupations, and lifestyle interrupted my academic goals. More recently, with us nearing retirement, the financial strain of rising tuition was a major drawback.

"Why don't you just jump in and do it?" Lee said that night at the kitchen table. "After all, it's not going to cost you anything, except time and work."

So, sizzling with trepidation, I went to late registration, the day before the first semester began. My head spun from the swiftness of it all. Then, I was gripped by a devil-may-care attitude. I couldn't feel any lower, so why not go for it? My advisor told me what courses I needed to complete my requirements.

"Math." The word slid from my mouth flat and distasteful—my old nemesis. Aside from all the legitimate reasons, it was one hurdle that stopped me short of my prize each time. Somewhere along life's path, my brain had computed me "numbers-challenged."

I have this little compulsion that insists I finish everything that I begin. All through the years, that little voice kept accusing, "you didn't get your degree." Sitting there in the advisor's office, it screamed, "it's now or never!"

A burst of do-or-die recklessness shot through me and I heard myself say, "sign me up for the Thinking Mathematically course." By golly, I'd do it or die trying.

After adding a required English course, my advisor suggested I stop there since I was just getting my feet wet after the long sabbatical. I took his advice and left, committed to six hours of credits.

Again, reality slammed me and my courage panicked. Imagine, me, who can't balance a checkbook, going into the numbers battle with a feather duster. Me, who could hardly drag myself out of bed some days, not to mention the mind-fog.

Disgusted, the "overcomer" me called the other me a "wimp" and I armed myself with a dozen #2 pencils and plenty of good erasers.

Those first days of classes tried me. Some days, I left Math class feeling I just might make it. Other days, I was certain I could never do it. I'd rush to the hospital ICU and see Mom, who had not yet come "back" to us. Then I would go home and study the new problems. Dizziness attacked me periodically as I struggled to see patterns in the numbers and symbols.

And then a strange thing happened. There's something about

taking charge of your life that spurs a domino effect of affirmative things. Kicking out compulsive things that ate up my time and energy, then replacing them with good, positive areas of aspiration boosted my self-confidence.

Another thing happened. I noticed my energy was near normal. I no longer had the debilitating incidents of lethargy and fatigue.

Yet — as my first math test approached, years doubts dogged me. Give up, give up, they insisted. You can't do it!

Mom transferred to Restorative Care, still critical. But now, I didn't have time to linger over any negative thoughts of her slow recovery. I developed patience.

The week of the test, nerves attacked me, making me dizzy with apprehension. On the morning of the exam, I went to the Math tutoring lab, where I'd spent many hours with my "Dream Team," headed by my Math teacher, Professor Kakaras, aided by Chris and Matt. When I left, with an hour to go before the test, I went to sit in the stillness of my car, listening to soft music and praying.

"Lord, you know how very much I want to succeed. Please — just give me peace. I've done all I can do to prepare. Now, I give myself into your hands. Just give me peace and calm as I face this test."

By the time I entered the classroom, the dizziness was gone.

Tranquility settled over me as I began working the problems. All I had studied came back to me. My mind was clear and focused. For the first time ever, numbers and symbols didn't confuse and scatter my focus. I was the last student to leave the classroom but that was okay. I finished all the problems.

I walked out into the warm sunshine and it hit me. This was a lifeline God tossed to me.

Going back to college resurrected my mind.

It resurrected me.

At the hospital, Mom said my name and squeezed my hand.

Life is good.

~Emily Sue Harvey

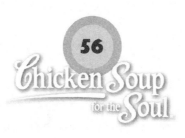

56

Finding Financial Freedom

The road leading to a goal does not separate you from the destination;
it is essentially a part of it.
~Charles DeLint

My wife, Amy was just about at the end of her rope. She'd been taking care of our finances for years, ever since the day I freaked out when there seemed to be so little money for so many bills. That was nearly fifteen years ago. Now, Amy had taken on her mother's affairs when she moved to an assisted living facility a hundred miles from our town.

By January 2008, the time had come for me to step up and take part of the load off my wife. Since I'd last paid the monthly bills, on-line banking had been created, and I found that made the task much easier. Amy sat me down and went over the monthly bills, and I discovered that our money situation had improved over the years. Still, we had some concerns about what we owed. One was a monthly payment for a line of credit loan we'd used. The money had gone to build a porch that ran along the front of our house and wrapped around the south end. We'd also bought a late model truck for me. Altogether, we owed close to $45,000 on that line of credit.

One of the first things I did when bill paying became my responsibility was to make a resolution that this loan would be paid off by the end of summer. And with that I set out a plan to make the promise come true. For one thing, I worked for an educational products company on a part-time basis and received monthly payments from them. That money went into the "kitty."

I also worked another job as a freelance writer for the local paper. Earnings from that work also went into the pot.

Plans were in the works for my retirement at the end of the school year in May. I'd taught high school English for thirty years, and at the age of fifty-six, the time had come to pursue other interests and let the next generation of teachers take over. At the beginning of the year, the system for which I worked had agreed to pay teachers $100 for each accumulated sick day they had at retirement. By the time taxes were carved out, I was left with about $5,000; another hunk of cash to go toward the effort.

We also deposited any leftover money we had at the end of each month. Our biggest single chunk of change came when I sold the truck we'd purchased a couple of years earlier. I returned to driving my old Nissan Pathfinder. I had driven it since 1987 and it still worked just fine.

Through the winter months and into spring, Amy and I squirreled away every extra penny we could find. Plans for a vacation in Charleston, South Carolina, fell by the wayside—another casualty of our determination to pay off this huge debt.

Summer came, and we continued to work on the debt. Each month we looked at the account we'd opened to see the cash amount grow. My resolution at times turned into an obsession, and at those times, Amy called me to account and insisted that I remain calm and logical.

Disappointment set in when we failed to reach our goal of paying off the debt by the end of summer. Still needing a bit more money, I fretted about whether we should pay off the bill at all. Maybe we should hold onto the cash for a while. Amy reminded me of the promise we'd made to each other, and that returned me to what our purpose had been over the previous months.

At the end of September, our account held enough money to pay off the debt. I again second-guessed the decision to pay off the loan; watching $45,000 disappear with a single stroke on the keyboard was scary. We took a deep breath, hit that key, and lifted a financial albatross from our necks.

For a day or so, I wondered whether or not our decision was a wise one. Then things hit the financial fan in America. Banks failed. Insurance giants needed billions to bail them out. The stock market plummeted, with record daily losses. Amy and I breathed easier not having to fork out a wad of cash on a monthly loan. It felt good to own the porch that we'd built.

Over the years, I've made plenty of resolutions. For years I quit smoking on New Year's Eve and celebrated the decision the next morning with a cup of coffee and a cigarette. More times than I can count, resolutions to lose weight have been sabotaged by such things as a meat lover's pizza and a six-pack of beer. This one time in my life, however, I made a resolution and kept it. The result was a sense of financial peace in our household in the midst of a time of economic upheaval.

~Joe Rector

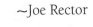

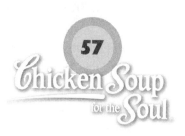

57

Chicken Soup
for the Soul

Overcoming Shyness

Worry and fear never rob tomorrow of its sorrow,
they only sap today of its joy.
~Leo Buscaglia

I was a shy kid. To me, people were complex, intimidating, unpredictable, and unknown. I didn't even like to answer the telephone for fear I'd have to talk to somebody I didn't know. I enjoyed the solitude of exploring the golden California hills that were near my home. Winding along hills and streams was invigorating yet peaceful.

However, at school I had to spend all day in the company of others. My escape was reading. Reading was acceptable and it was solitary. Studying was another thing I could do quietly and by myself. I spent a lot of time studying and was rewarded with good grades. My one downfall was Spanish—I'd get all As on my written work and tests, but Ds and Fs on the spoken part. I simply could not get up in front of the class to speak those simple dialogues.

Eventually I went to college. I realized that some people were rather fun to hang out with. Yet my childhood shyness carried over and I found myself tongue-tied and embarrassed whenever I found myself in a conversation.

During my third year of college, I decided that I'd had enough of being shy. I found that I enjoyed being around people and I wanted to be able to converse freely like the other students around me. I resolved to change my outlook and behavior and overcome my shyness.

Along the way, I had learned a few words and phrases in several foreign languages — Spanish, German, and Russian. One day while on campus, I noticed an advertisement for positions on the local classical music radio station. I had grown up listening to classical music, and I loved it. I also realized that my language background enabled me to easily pronounce names such as Tchaikovsky, Albinoni, Chopin, Dvorak, and Rachmaninov.

In order to get a job at the radio station, applicants needed to submit an audition tape and be interviewed. My goal was merely to survive the interview and making the tape — going into a recording booth and reading advertisements and announcing symphonies and operas. I had absolutely no background in radio, and absolutely no hope of getting the job. The idea of talking to thousands of listeners in "radioland" terrified me. No, I didn't really want the job, I just wanted to know that I could speak onto a tape and talk to an interviewer.

I survived the interview. The station manager was soft spoken and had a wonderful mellow voice that made me feel calm and comfortable. The recording booth was a bit intimidating with all the gauges, buttons and flashing lights, but it was intriguing as well. I was given brief descriptions of symphonies and a public service announcement to read, and a list of composers' names to pronounce.

It wasn't hard to read the descriptions and announcements, and the names, long familiar to me, were simple to speak. I left the recording session with a sense of relief that it was over, and a sense of accomplishment that I had actually done this strange and terrifying thing.

I was even more terrified to discover, about two weeks later, that I had actually landed the job. I was to work part time, at night and on weekends. I had to sit in the on-air studio, play recordings, and talk to thousands of unknown people throughout the state of Utah! I learned, too, that Saturday afternoons featured a listener request time. That meant I had to answer the phone and talk to people; noting, finding, and playing their requests.

It was a challenging job, but I grew to enjoy it immensely. I announced music to thousands of listeners in Salt Lake City and throughout Utah. In addition to announcing music and taking requests, I held contests, awarding free tickets "to the third caller." I recorded and aired public service and promotional announcements. I began to feel comfortable talking to these people, these strangers, who I couldn't even see.

It was a unique experience, being a DJ. After a few months, I realized that talking to people was not scary, but actually fun. I married and had five children. Speaking to people and navigating bureaucracy became simple. Eventually I found myself in another job—interviewing people and writing their stories in a weekly community newspaper.

Although I now spend many hours each week talking with people, I'm still basically a quiet person. Perhaps it is my soft voice and my quiet nature that helps draw people out as they respond to my questions as I interview them. My former shyness is an asset, as I can relate to people who feel discomfort when they talk to this local newspaper reporter. I still enjoy moments of solitude and the peace found in nature. But I'm also glad I resolved to make a change in my life that has opened many doors and opportunities that I never knew existed.

~Linda Butler

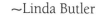

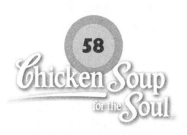

58

My Triumph in a Taxi

Panic is a sudden desertion of us,
and a going over to the enemy of our imagination.
~Christian Nevell Bovee

"You can do this," my husband said, as we were about to get into the back of a New York City cab.

"No, Bob. I can't. I've made a million resolutions to conquer my fear. Not once have they worked."

We were standing in line outside Penn Station. Taxis pulled up, one after another in a whirlwind and whisked everyone, including the women and children, away.

As our turn in purgatory approached, I thought, "I'm going to have a panic attack in the cab, and (here's the important part) I won't be able to handle it."

I have the same problem that lots of people have in elevators, dentist offices and airplanes—the fear of the fear.

I continued my, "No, I can't!" thinking. I imagined myself in the tiny space in the back seat with my huge suitcase on my lap smushed up against my face so I'd suffocate. "This figures," I thought to myself. "All this time I've assumed I'd die in an airplane. Instead, I'll be snuffed out by a Samsonite."

Of course, purely because of what I was telling myself, my body systems began to sky-rocket into a full flight or fight panic response.

"Breathe," Bob said.

"I am," I said defensively. "I'm just not breathing out."

"Breathe," he repeated. "And focus."

"I'm not having a baby, Bob!" I screamed. "I'm having a panic attack."

I thought, "What on earth made me make this stupid resolution again?"

There were only three families in front of us in line. I told the couple behind us to take our place. I kept doing this with other passengers, until I calmed down. Now, that was not magically going to happen unless I changed my "this is impossible" negative self-talk.

I looked toward the streets. I saw maniacal taxi drivers careening around curves, missing other cars by a hair. All the while our turn in line was coming closer.

And then, there we were, facing the steel beast. The driver began putting our luggage in the trunk. I looked at the tiny back seat, saw the metal grate separating passengers from the driver and said, "Can I sit in front?" I figured I'd be less claustrophobic.

"Does a disability prevent you from sitting in the back?"

"I'm neurotic."

"Sorry."

"You can do this," Bob said again, as we were about to get in the back of the cab.

"No, I can't." And just that one sentence put the lid on my courage.

And so, as you can probably guess, I had finally given up on my resolve. We started to walk the eight blocks to our hotel. I was filled with self hatred. "I'm tossing this resolution out the window. I will never conquer my fear."

I started to cry as we lumbered with our suitcases down the crowded avenue. I was a pathetic sight; tears dripping down my face. I stopped and put my bags down. "Wait," I said to Bob. Not realizing I had been crying, he stopped and looked at me with anguish on his face. "It's okay," he said, wiping my cheek with his fingers.

"No. It's not. Everybody in the world can get in to a cab but me."

I watched as cabs sped by, knowing they were forever off-limits to me. And that's when the miracle and the magic happened. Bob, always mysteriously simpatico, put his arm around my shoulder. "Everybody's afraid of something," he said. He saw me eyeing the cabs. "You don't have to do it, but if you wanted to, how would you pull it off?"

"Well, the biggest thing is that I made a resolution to finally, no matter what, conquer this. That itself is what's most motivating." Then I tried to remember what had worked a little for me in the past. "I'd tell myself that anxiety symptoms feel terrible but they won't last." He nodded encouragingly. Now I was on a roll. I pictured myself in the taxi, not necessarily in a calm state, because I knew realistically that was not likely to happen this time. Instead I saw myself looking out the window, feeling anxious, but (and this is the important part) knowing I could handle it. I wasn't going to go crazy or have a heart attack or whatever my fill-in-the-blank terror would be.

Becoming calm wasn't necessarily my goal for now. Doing what I wanted in spite of and along with my fear was.

I wanted to hail a cab. I took one step toward the sidewalk. The prickly heat of tension covered my arms. I stopped. "I'm not letting you win," I growled silently to my demons. I took two more venturing steps ahead. I forced my arm in the air and a cab slowed down. My knees lost most of their strength but they still held me up.

I turned back. With my eyes, I pleaded for Bob to take over, somehow.

We often read each other's minds. "I can't do it for you," he said. "It has to be your victory."

And with the hard steel look of an Olympian sprinter poised in the ready, I heard the starter gun go off in my head. With my level of terror only matched by my level of determination to resolve my problem, I raised my arm. The cab stopped.

I opened the door quickly before I could talk myself out of it. "I am doing this come heck or high water or anything you want to throw at me, you lousy panic monster!" The symptoms came on like a rushing army. "I can tolerate it," I thought. My heart pounded. I began to tremble. "Nothing's going to happen," I said like a mantra.

"These sensations can't hurt me. You've felt them a hundred times before. Breathe from your diaphragm; long deep breaths to the slow rhythmic count of four. That will take you down. Just wait it out."

"I can't handle this!" I began to think.

"Don't listen in," I said back to myself. "Concentrate on your breathing. It's only an adrenaline rush and I promise it will pass." And then I added, with a loving whisper to my frightened brave soul, "I am so very proud of you."

We made it to the hotel. For the entire ride I had given myself "yes, you can" messages.

And they worked!

I celebrated my life-changing accomplishment in my usual sophisticated manner: room service. We polished off Buffalo wings, brie on bruschetta, some sort of seafood in a dreamy cream sauce and four Napoleons.

Now, lots of people might not think it takes courage to get into a cab. Not compared to scaling a mountain or speaking in front of two hundred people. But it's all the same. I believe everything in this life is what we make of it in our hearts and our heads and therefore our actions.

If we panic in supermarket lines or airplanes or driving over bridges or in crowded malls and are able to muster the courage to proceed, even for just a tiny part of the way, then we are medal-deserving Olympian heroes, in every sense of the word.

The finish line has nothing to do with crossing that line or the having the fastest time. It's taking that first trembling step.

~Saralee Perel

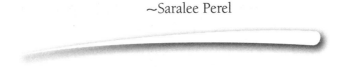

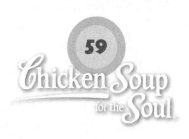

59

Taking Taekwondo

Find something that you love and go for it!
~Author Unknown

When I was twenty-six years old, my left lung collapsed. The surgeon who repaired the damage told me bluntly that I needed to quit smoking—I was at three packs a day—or I would die. I had been told this before, but the facts had never been this convincing. So I quit smoking—and grew heavier and grumpier by the day. I was terrified that I would eventually give in and start smoking again. But I knew that, once and for all, I had to take control of my health by getting in shape and eating right.

In the beginning it wasn't easy. I went for walks, but soon lost interest. I counted calories, but couldn't stop eating. I considered joining an aerobics class, but couldn't imagine myself prancing around with a bunch of strangers.

Then one day I walked by a building: New Horizons Black Belt Academy of Taekwondo. I didn't even pause. I walked right in and took my first lesson. I was too dizzy and out of breath to make it through the first class. But I knew I'd be back the next day, and the next, and the next—I'd fallen in love.

Immediately, I learned my body could do things I never thought possible. I practiced a Taekwondo "form," which is a pattern of movements almost like a dance. As I caught sight of myself in the mirror, I was struck by how beautiful the form was—and how beautiful I was. I had never thought of my body that way before.

Every Monday night, the instructor demonstrated self-defense techniques. One evening, she asked me to show the other white belts, my fellow beginners, how to do a technique. It was intoxicating. I'd been practicing for only a few weeks and I had already mastered something. I had achieved something physical—me—the playground klutz, the sideline spectator.

A few weeks later, I earned my yellow belt and began "sparring," a form of mock combat that involves kicking and punching other people, and getting kicked and punched back. At first, I couldn't hit anyone. Jeanne, a tall black belt, patiently coached me. She simply stood there, hands lowered, saying, "Okay, go ahead and hit me." I did so, timidly at first, then with mounting confidence, until one day I hit her hard enough to matter and she hugged me.

It wasn't the sort of thing that would make my mother proud, but it made me proud. It made Jeanne proud, too. I realized that I was worth defending.

Getting hit also frightened me. A punch or a kick didn't even have to touch me for me to flinch. But after enough practice I learned not to be afraid. I grew bolder, I hit harder, people hit me back just as hard, and I discovered a profound and electrifying truth: You could get hit, you could get hit hard, and it didn't have to demoralize you. You didn't have to fall down and cry, or wait for a man to come along and rescue you. You could take it, smile, and defend yourself.

Years later, after I earned my black belt, I visited a new physician for my annual exam, and he said, "I see you've had rheumatoid arthritis for more than ten years, but you seem to be getting around okay."

I grinned. Oh, boy. "I can do a jump spinning-wheel kick to your head," I wanted to say, but did not. "Yeah," I said, instead. "I do all right."

~Jennifer Lawler

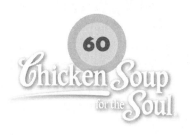

60

The Last Time

> *To cease smoking is the easiest thing I ever did.*
> *I ought to know because I've done it a thousand times.*
> ~Mark Twain

My hand quivered as I held my lover for the last time. Our relationship, twenty turbulent years in the making, was coming to an end. I had said goodbye countless times before. I prayed this time it was for real.

The two of us were rarely seen apart. Even when we couldn't be close, I counted the minutes until our joyful reunion. Those close to me tried to make me see how destructive this behavior was and if I had been honest with myself from the beginning, I would have had to agree. But when you're young and foolish, reason has no place in such decisions.

Now, twenty years later, I prayed that this goodbye would be our last. I sat in the cold watching the last moments, then the last seconds, slip quietly away. No words were spoken. No tears shed. This was my moment of anguished victory to relish alone. In a few months, maybe a few years, I would celebrate. But right now I needed to be strong, though a fragile strength it was.

I told no one. I proceeded as if nothing had happened. I needed time to heal—perhaps a very long time. I had learned from past attempts at independence that well-meaning friends offering support and encouragement served only to threaten the delicate balance I struggled to maintain until I could learn to live on my own. Their suggestions would only prick at the painful wound I was desperately trying to close as quickly as possible.

"I'm done," I finally said.

"Yeah, me too. I'm going to bed." My husband pulled the cigarette from his lips and snubbed it out in the ashtray, completely unaware of the monumental turning point my life had just experienced. "Luv you. Sleep sweet."

I had not told even him that I was going to smoke my last cigarette on that evening. Even if I had, he, like everyone else, would have smiled and said, "That's great, babe. Good luck." Then he would walk away knowing that the next time he saw me, the Marlboro man and I would have found our way back to each other once again. My frequent attempts to quit had become a running joke among those who knew me.

I sat alone in the garage and stared at the littered ashtray. It was December 30th of 2003. It was my New Year's resolution—the same one I had made countless times before. Year after year, it would be the same story. I would slip after a day or two, then console myself by saying, "Next birthday or next anniversary or next whatever." It was so much easier to quit on the next "whatever" than it was on this "whatever."

As with all smokers, I had a long list of reasons to quit. Health, money, and a growing social stigma were among them. However, unlike most smokers, I had the unfortunate experience of watching my mother die from lung cancer up close and personal.

I can still remember sitting in the hospital room day after day watching them suction chunks of black and brown lung tissue through a tube that was inserted through her nose and down into her chest. I would hold her hand and pray for the strength not to pass out or scream in terror at the sight. When it was over, I would race down to the parking garage and suck down two cigarettes as quickly as I could, trying to numb the pain.

I still remember her asking me, "You don't smoke, do you? You see what it's done to me!" She could only form words with her lips. Her voice had been silenced by the barrage of tubes being forced down her throat and wind pipe.

"No Mom, I don't smoke," I lied. The betrayal was almost more than I could bear.

She died when I was twenty-two. One would think that experience would make me swear off tobacco forever. It didn't. I continued to smoke for another eighteen years.

I tried using the twelve steps of AA that had worked so beautifully to help me get sober. No luck. I tried patches and gum, sometimes at the same time. I tried meditation, medication, rationing, writing farewell letters to my cigarettes (that was weird!), eating licorice, sucking cinnamon sticks. I attended classes, counseling, church.

It was as if God was saying, "You're on your own, kid."

On that dark December night, it was just me and those cigarettes. Then God decided to step in. I had an epiphany. He hit me where it hurt most—my pride. It dawned on me that I had been sucker punched by the tobacco companies and they were laughing all the way to the bank! If there's one thing I hate, it's being made a fool of.

Now I was mad. No more "Farewell, my love." Now it was, "Leave me alone, you bastard!" Anger is a powerful force.

I was truly done.

I didn't throw my last pack away. In fact, I carried it and a lighter with me for about two months. Maybe it was that need for an escape—I've always been a bit commitment-phobic. Maybe it was to prove that I was more powerful than the cigarettes. Maybe it was to spite the tobacco companies by showing them I had truly won. But I never again slid out one of those slender white daggers from their hiding place.

Four and a half years later, I can tell you that it was, along with getting sober, the best decision I ever made. My life today is different in so many ways I would need a hundred pages to list them all. I feel better, sleep better, look better, smell better, food tastes better. My hair is healthy, my skin is clear, my nails are white again, my teeth are white again.

I would be lying if I said there weren't moments that a cigarette would taste really good. All I have to do is think it through the same way I do a drink. Do I really want to deal again with the ball and chain that's on the other side? Smoking is a physical, mental and emotional addiction—every bit as powerful as alcohol or drugs. It is still amazing to me how something that weighs less than an ounce was such a heavy load in my life for so long.

As I reflect on my smoke-free years, I can truly say I have had some of the best times of my life. Precious moments and happy occasions are no longer overshadowed and interrupted by my compulsion to find a hiding place to indulge my addiction. I can finally live in the moment.

I still have challenges and disappointments because they are a fact of life. But instead of being overwhelmed and retreating to the dulling effects of a cigarette, I have the confidence and energy to overcome whatever obstacles come my way.

And those victories come with their own brand of happiness that I could have never known before.

~Stacy Murphy

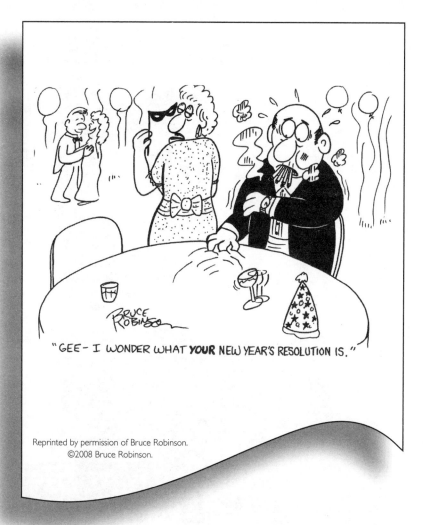

"GEE - I WONDER WHAT *YOUR* NEW YEAR'S RESOLUTION IS."

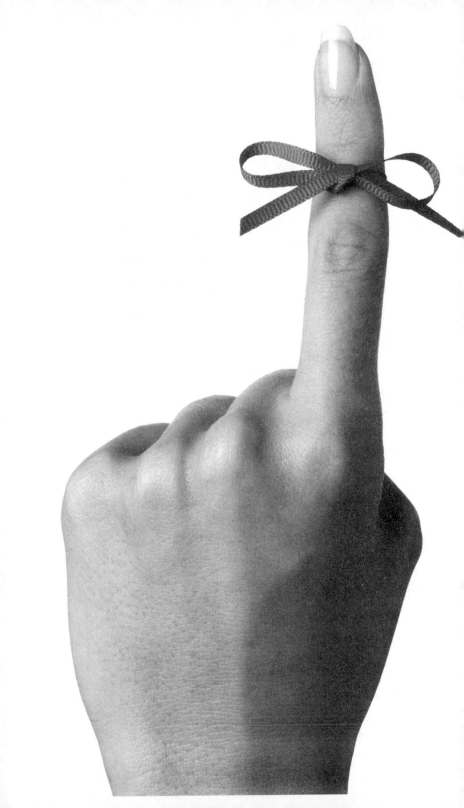

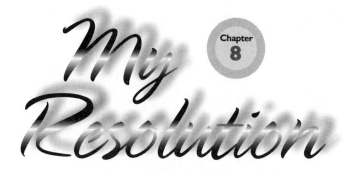

My Resolution

Chapter
8

Gotta Laugh!

*At the height of laughter,
the universe is flung into a kaleidoscope of new possibilities.*

~Jean Houston

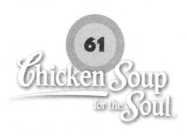

61

Dirty Socks and Carbon Footprints

I think the environment should be put in the category of our national security.
Defense of our resources is just as important as defense abroad.
Otherwise what is there to defend?
~Robert Redford

Global warming is probably the most serious issue affecting our planet. Although I suspect if we all simply stopped driving our kids to soccer, the Earth would plummet into another Ice Age. So this year, in addition to boycotting my son's away games, my goal is to take additional steps to reduce carbon emissions, conserve energy, and keep the ice caps intact. I figure that if I reduce my family's impact on the Earth, not only will I help the environment, I might even improve my own quality of life.

In my quest for carbon neutrality, I've decided to stop vacuuming. Turns out, a canister vacuum like mine sucks up a whopping 800 watts of electricity per month. Now, the cat hair on the couch and the dust bunnies under the dining room table can provide extra insulation as well as visible proof that I am doing my part for the planet. When company comes, I'll just unscrew our fluorescent bulbs (more energy savings!) and light a candle. I'm sure my guests will appreciate the ambiance.

With the time I save by not vacuuming, I can relax and watch television (which consumes a mere 180 watts a month). Who knew that tuning into *Oprah* and the *Food Network* could help stave off global warming?

To further reduce my family's carbon footprint, I've also cut way back on how frequently I do laundry. After all, in a month of average use (and my family is way above average) the washing machine drains about 15,000 gallons of potable water, as well as more than 600 watts of electricity and the dryer burns up a staggering 13,000 watts.

So when the kids say, "Moooommmmm, I don't have any clean socks!" I just say, "Turn them inside out and they'll be good for another week." Same goes for underwear. I know Al Gore would approve and I feel good about treading lightly (albeit in dirty knee-highs) on the Earth.

Deforestation also contributes to climate change. We all know that saving paper saves trees. So, in the spirit of environmental consciousness, I've replaced the rolls of squeezable Charmin in my kids' bathroom with those little, gray, scratchy sheets that they have at highway rest stops. I lost the ability to control their toilet paper consumption when they stopped demanding, "Wipe me!" Now, unsupervised, they gaily unfurl yards of the stuff at each sitting. I know—because I'm the only one whoever replaces the empty rolls, and I replace them frequently. The result of this ticker-tape mentality has resulted in clear cutting in Brazil and clogged drains in my bathroom. Maybe the little scratchy sheets will make using toilet paper a little less of a celebratory occasion and more of an opportunity to meditate on the importance of trees. They're lucky I don't put a basket of oak leaves next to the toilet.

Perhaps the most significant step I've taken to stop global warming is to cut my consumption of gasoline. I've simply reduced the number of unnecessary car trips to places like... the supermarket.

The way I see it, if we're out of milk, the kids can drink water. If we're out of food, we can get take-out. Ordering Chinese food or pizza saves some of the 12,500 watts that the stove uses during an average month and because the delivery guy's out there driving around anyway, I figure he might as well stop at my house. When

I do cook, I try to use the microwave (only 1,300 watts!) instead of the range. That means when the kids ask, "What's for dinner?" the answer is popcorn.

I feel good that my family is doing more to help protect our planet. Personally, I think laying off the housework can really make a difference. The way I figure it, sometimes doing more means doing way less—and that's a sacrifice I am happy to make.

~Carol Band

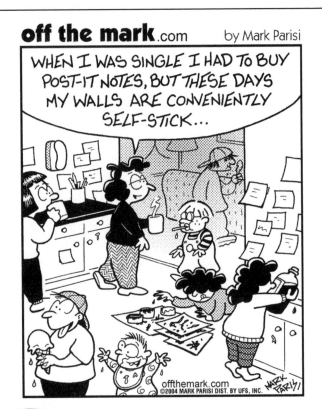

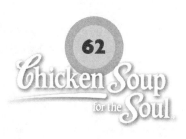

You Say You Want a Resolution

Yesterday, everybody smoked his last cigar, took his last drink and swore his last oath. Today, we are an exemplary community. Thirty days from now, we shall have cast our reformation to the winds and forgotten our resolutions.

~Mark Twain

I do not like New Year's resolutions. What happens at the stroke of midnight on New Year's Eve that suddenly makes the person you were last year so bad that you have to spend an entire year working to change yourself?

Of course, having said that, you must know that even though I hate New Year's resolutions, I do actually write them. I don't know why. I think it's peer pressure. My friends do it, so I must also do it. Now that I think about it, it's exactly that attitude that got me into a lot of trouble in high school.

So you'd think I'd have learned my lesson by now; after all I've been out of high school for twen—um, ten years or so. But no, I haven't. Sadly, I continue to try to reinvent myself every year. But this year I was determined to do something different, to not give in to peer pressure.

So this year, instead of my resolutions, I did some research and found the top ten New Year's resolutions. And once I found them I figured, why not use them? After all, everybody else does or they wouldn't be the top ten, right? Yes, I know I'm giving in to peer pressure again, but I just can't help it. Some habits are hard to break.

1. Lose weight.
    Sadly, I will never accomplish this resolution because I love food. And it loves me so much that it sticks to my butt and never leaves no matter how much dieting I do.

2. Stop smoking.
    Done! Wow, that was easier than I thought. I just accomplished a resolution with no effort whatsoever. Of course, I don't actually smoke, but still, it was on the list, and I am absolutely not smoking. So it must count, right?

3. Stick to a budget.
    I'm not sure exactly what that budget thing is, but I resolve to actually make sure I have money in the checking account before I spend it. You know, this is going to be a tough resolution to conquer, but I think I can do it. Maybe.

4. Save more money.
    What does save mean? Does it mean buy more stuff on sale? I can do that. In fact, I've already accomplished this resolution several times this week. And I plan to accomplish it even more after next payday. After all, I am on a budget now.

5. Find a better job.
    Oh, please. What's better than motherhood? I mean, where else could I find a job that involves driving, arguing, shopping, food preparation, house cleaning, teaching, and entertainment management and not get paid? Hmm. Maybe there's something to this resolution after all.

6. Become more organized.
    This is the resolution that frightens me the most. I am a terminally disorganized person. I love stuff. I can't throw away anything. I have Junior's baby bibs, for Pete's sake.

They're stained and stinky and I keep them because how on earth could I just toss them out in the trash? They're treasured pieces of my baby's history. I know... I know. I need help.

7. Exercise more.
    One more resolution done. I just walked from the den to the kitchen to get a piece of chocolate. That's more exercise than I've done in weeks. And of course, putting the chocolate in my mouth counts as an arm curl. Or whatever that exercise is called.

8. Be more patient at work/with others.
    What? Are you kidding me? I am so patient, I define patient. I just dare you to find a more patient person than me. Well, hurry up, I'm waiting. Oh, you can't find one, can you? Ahem. Maybe I could use a little work in this area.

9. Eat better.
    Fine. From now on, I will order the Filet-O-Fish instead of the Big Mac. After all, fish is better for me than red meat.

10. Become a better person.
    Well, heck, how vague is that? Become better at what? Empathy? Tennis? Beating up my neighbor? Gee whiz. Some specifics would be nice.

Well, there you have them, a list of the top ten resolutions that I found. I don't know how many I can do—but you can bet I'll try. I'm signing up for tennis lessons right after I finish my fried fish sandwich and hit the sale racks at Target.

~Laurie Sontag

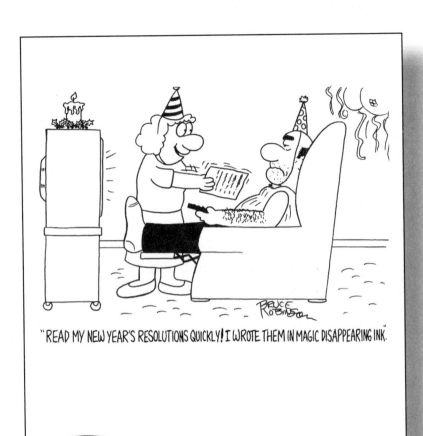

"READ MY NEW YEAR'S RESOLUTIONS QUICKLY! I WROTE THEM IN MAGIC DISAPPEARING INK."

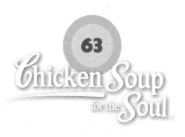

The Great Pillow Caper

A ruffled mind makes a restless pillow.
~Charlotte Brontë

Not as noble as feeding the hungry perhaps, but my New Year's resolution was to buy a new pillow. It wouldn't bring world peace, but my pillow was flat! Humans spend six to eight hours a day sleeping, or not, because of the comfort of their pillow. I was losing sleep over mine. A new one would improve my physical and mental health. Plus as resolutions go, it was easy to accomplish, or so I thought.

Of course my husband Dan needed one too. He thought that I would just get one for each of us. Wrong! Money problems are touted as the major failure of marriages. I think it could be the wrong pillow selection by one spouse for the other. I wasn't taking that chance. Besides, Dan really needed to get out more in the real world of retail. Sure he shops on Christmas Eve as a bonding experience with our kids Chris and Sarah. He likes to linger in the big box hardware "we've got everything you need for your home and workshop" stores. In reality he has no clue what's out there and what things cost.

There was the time he decided to buy new sheets. Not knowing that that they were priced by the piece he took his selections to the cashier thinking he would be paying around $40. When the cost totaled $120, Sarah, who was with him, said he turned white as a... sheet. Embarrassed, he completed the transaction figuring that I could return them. They were the most expensive sheet I ever owned

Off I dragged him to our local bed and bath store to check out the selection. Right inside the door was a bin full of pillows — two to the pack for $7.99. "Well that was easy," he remarked.

"No way!" I exclaimed. "There is a better selection in the middle of the store."

As we rounded the corner, his eyes glazed over as towers of gleaming white pillows rose to tremendous heights.

High on the wall, a huge sign described in minutiae how to pick out a pillow. Dan is an engineer and loves the details. I figured this would distract him for a while and prevent him from hyperventilating. As we stood there gazing up at the sign, I had the strangest feeling that someone had joined us.

"So what are we staring at?" asked my friends Terry and Terry.

Terry P., the joker of the two, claimed that he had had the same pillow for twelve years. He started into a stand-up pillow talk comedy routine. By now our section of this usually quiet store was getting crowded. Who knew so many people had resolved to buy a new pillow? A woman across the aisle pretending to study a memory foam pillow was obviously chuckling at Terry's monologue.

While Dan provided straight lines for Terry P., Terry M. and I got serious about checking out the pillows. A sign on the shelf asked, "Do you sleep on your side or back?" "Yes" we said in unison.

"Here's one made from down," he observed. "Who would pay $95 for a pillow? If you don't like it will they let you bring it back?" I immediately flashed back to a childhood memory of an old *Dick Van Dyke* episode. A con artist sold Laura "down" pillows. The whole group buried their faces and snorted the pillows trying to figure out what the odd smell was emanating from them. They were filled with chicken feathers. In a funny, feather-flying scene Dick represents himself in court to try to get his money back.

Dan can't understand how I remember these things. It's because my head isn't clogged with all those tedious technical details.

Next to the down pillows were pillows with 500-thread count covers. 500-thread count? How does that improve the comfort of a pillow? A high thread count in sheets makes them softer (see reference to the $120 sheets in paragraph three), but I myself always use a pillowcase. Could I feel those 500-threads through the 600-count pillowcase? If my pillowcase is only 100-count will the total equal the pleasure of a 600-count? Maybe it is a special sleep aid. If you can't sleep, count threads instead of counting sheep—1 thread, 2 threads, 3 threads... zzzzzzzzzzzzzzzzzzzzzzzzz.

The crowd now resembled a sleepover. We shared bedtime stories. Mine was about Joe, who always brought his own beat-up, contoured-to-his head pillow wherever he went. Joe became ill on a trip to Canada. In his delirious state, he somehow left his pillow behind. How would he ever get a good night's sleep again? His wife contacted the hotel. After many phone calls meticulously describing the pillow and much negotiation the hotel agreed to send it. After paying fees and shipping, the bill was outrageous. To make matters worse, they sent the wrong pillow!

Terry and Terry picked out allergen-free pillow protectors and wandered around the store. A new guy came breezing in, store employee in tow. She showed him the inventory, explaining about pillows for side versus back sleepers and which one she personally used. Those of us in the crowd, now resembling the Verizon Wireless network, shuffled inconspicuously close enough to hear the scoop. In the end he grabbed a pillow without even looking at it from the $12.99 bin. Obviously thinking himself too cool for the party, he went on his way. Well, he was no help!

I finally picked out a pillow by taking several around the store trying them on things that might simulate an actual bed rather than a metal shelf. Dan picked one from the same bin as the cool guy. Purchases in hand we left the party before the pizzas arrived, said goodbye to the Terrys and went on our way.

That night, when Dan took his pillow out of the plastic, it inflated like a giant balloon in the Macy's Thanksgiving Day Parade. His head was about a foot above mine. After the laughter subsided, I nestled into my own new pillow.

It took me several nights to get a good sleep—I had a cold and couldn't breathe. The first morning I found myself slobbering all over my new pillow—so that's why you can't return them! Even Dick Van Dyke wouldn't defend me. When I finally slept well, I think it was a direct result of the nighttime cold medication.

After it was all said and done, my great pillow caper provided more benefit than I ever could have imagined. I enjoyed a good laugh, relived childhood memories, spent time with friends, preserved my marriage, and my health was better from getting enough sleep. Hey, what percentage of the rest of the world can say that they successfully accomplished their New Year's resolution and more?

~Linda Ruddy

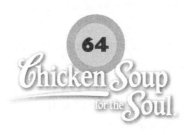

Be Prepared... for Anything!

If you must reread old love letters, better pick a room without mirrors.
~Mignon McLaughlin

Let's face it... I'm a pack rat of the worst kind. An incurable romantic, I save corks from champagne bottles, dried gardenias from the junior prom, a torn theater ticket from *Oklahoma*. But most revered of all are those letters I've collected from my travels around the world... not always written in the best English, but all the more charming for their sentiments, even those that are nearly indecipherable.

So you can imagine the heart-rending task that faced me when I made a resolution to downsize to smaller quarters and get rid of all unnecessary "junk" from the past fifty years. Disposing of furniture? Dishes? Clothing? Exhausting, but entirely feasible. But disposing of old love letters? Devastating!

As I sat on the floor of my bedroom, removing each letter from its fragile envelope, I relived a lifetime of Robert Browning wanna-bes, savoring every tender phrase, every delicately turned declaration.

Then I gathered the bundles of these ancient treasures and reluctantly placed them in a garbage can by the roadside.

I stood at the kitchen sink washing dishes when sudden activity in the street caught my eye.

Three youngsters in khaki uniforms rode their bicycles back and forth in front of my house. Precious little lambs. What were they up to? Some kind of collection for the Boy Scouts? Wait a minute! They had dropped their bikes on my front lawn. They were approaching my garbage can! What in heaven's name were they doing? One lifted the lid, and the others were reaching in and rummaging through... my love letters! They were removing them by the handfuls and stuffing them in their knapsacks.

Screaming like a banshee, I raced out the kitchen door. "What do you think you're doing?" I screeched.

"We're earning our stamp-collecting merit badges," smiled one lad sweetly.

"Put those letters back this very minute!" I bellowed.

"But these are neat stamps. Some are fifty years old!"

"I have a better idea," I said cunningly. "Why don't we gather them all up and take them to the barbecue pit in our backyard and have a marshmallow roast?"

"What about our stamp collecting badges?"

"Isn't there a marshmallow badge?"

The boys looked dubious. "We were going to sell the ones we don't want at the Boy Scout yard sale," said one. "We're earning a trip to Sea World."

"And what is purple prose going for these days?" I muttered under my breath. "Whatever happened to cookie sales?"

The boys glared. "Those are for Girl Scouts!"

"How many tickets to Sea World do you need?"

"Three."

I did a quick calculation and recoiled in shock. $59.95 times three... $179.85! But compared to having all the mothers of the Scout troop reading fifty years of my love letters?

I bit the bullet. "Can I write you a check?"

Which only goes to show you that love letters in the sand are a whole lot cheaper than those in the trash.

~Phyllis W. Zeno

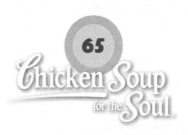

"Cold Turkey"

I don't have a problem with caffeine. I have a problem without caffeine!
~Author Unknown

Having worked the night shift for the past twelve years, I've become something of a coffee aficionado. Although I've always enjoyed a good cup of Joe, working from 10:30 P.M. to 7:00 A.M. has increased my appreciation of the hot energy-giving elixir exponentially. Drinking coffee all night long has helped me stay awake and work while most of the rest of the world is fast asleep.

Unfortunately, a slow, gradual build-up of all that caffeine often left me too wired to fall asleep during the day, or woke me up hours before my brain and body wanted to. After one restless sleep session too many, I resolved to give up my beloved Thermos of get-up-and-go. I would train my body to crave water instead of java and I was sure I'd be calmer, more peaceful, and would hopefully sleep a whole lot better.

There were other factors behind my decision. Every so often a report would pop up in the media claiming that coffee wasn't really all that good for a body. Of course, a few months later another report would state that coffee was actually beneficial. But I wanted to see how I'd feel without any artificial stimulants coursing through my veins. I wondered what it would be like to re-discover my own natural energy level instead of the caffeine inflated one I'd been coasting upon ever since I had my first cup of coffee back in college.

My wife suggested I wean myself off the bean gradually but I decided to go cold turkey. One Saturday morning I had my last cup of coffee before going outside to mow the front lawn.

This is going to be a piece of cake, I thought, as I made neat green swaths up and down the grass. I feel great and I'm going to feel even better. Who needs coffee?

My sense of well-being continued as the day went on. I did all my usual weekend chores with my usual amount of vim and vigor. After mowing the lawn, I swept out the garage, and washed the car. I did notice a slight headache forming behind my eyes as I rinsed soapsuds off the car, but by concentrating on how much better I was going to feel as soon as I was totally caffeine-free, I managed to ignore it.

Sunday morning, I awoke with an even bigger headache. Opening my eyes, I noticed that focusing on the alarm clock was a lot more challenging than usual. I also noticed that a distinct case of brain fog was forming as I struggled to remember what I planned on doing that day.

Let's see. Get up. Have breakfast. Read the paper. Go back to bed.

I had to do more than that but for the life of me, I couldn't remember. Stumbling out of the bedroom, I found my wife sitting at the kitchen table reading the paper and looking very bright eyed as she drank what was probably her fourth cup of coffee. Lifting her eyes, she gave me a long, appraising glance before returning to "Dear Abby."

"I told you that you should have weaned yourself off coffee instead of going cold turkey," she remarked. "How did you sleep last night?"

"Great," I mumbled. And I had slept well, a clear indication that my resolution was working.

"That's good," she said, "because you look terrible."

I was feeling terrible too, like I'd been dropped on my head into a giant bowl of pea soup. "I think I'll have a couple of aspirin," I announced. "I'm sure I'll feel better soon."

My wife poured herself another cup of coffee. "I'm sure you will," she agreed.

By the third day my headache was gone and I really did feel better. The brain fog had lifted and my energy level was assumedly as its natural set point.

That was the problem. Dragging myself through work that night, I discovered something: the natural set point for my energy level had apparently gotten lower and lower over the years. I now seemed to have enough energy to get up, eat, and go back to bed. Making it through the night shift caffeine-free was a lot like trying to make it through a maze wearing a blindfold. Not easy.

After one week of being caffeine-free, I slipped and had a cup of coffee at three in the morning. As the hot liquid hit my bloodstream I realized something: I missed my coffee. I didn't want to be caffeine-free. I wanted my old, artificial energy level back.

So I compromised. I drink half-decaf, half-full strength coffee now and I don't drink nearly as much as I used to. I'm able to sleep during the day and I'm able to do my job at night. My resolution didn't last too long but that's okay. I simply changed it from resolving to give up coffee to resolving to be a lot more thoughtful about how much coffee I drink. I'm paying closer attention to the signals my body gives out and I like to think that I'm a little healthier for the experiment.

One thing is for certain—the next time I make a resolution I'm going to listen to my wife and take it slowly. Cold turkey is best for sandwiches only.

~Mark Musolf

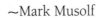

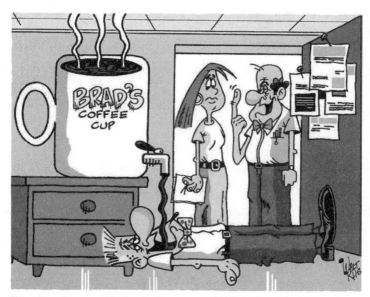

"Brad made a resolution to have only 'ONE CUP' of coffee a day!"

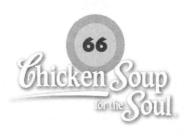

Resolutions for Sale

I have to exercise in the morning before my brain figures out what I'm doing.
~Marsha Doble

Friday mornings were a fun time for a group of us ladies who were new to the city. However, this particular Friday, I didn't feel well. I didn't go with the others for our usual all-day shopping and lunch date.

While driving to the grocery store, I noticed a huge amount of goods displayed on a lawn in front of a house. The sign intrigued me, so I stopped.

"Resolutions for SALE," was printed on a large sign.

Exercise equipment, mostly in the original boxes, filled the large yard. A variety of exercise clothing hung on a clothing rack. Several pairs of jogging shoes were still in the original boxes. Several shelves were filled with books and videos... each promising super results with a particular exercise routine.

As I walked through the maze of items, I read the notes taped to each one. Each note told a story:

Yes, I promised to have thighs like Suzanne Somers, but I'm too busy chasing kids around to master this routine.

My husband forgot he had bought this same treadmill last year, so both are brand new.

*Special price on this exercise bike. The noise from the wheel
makes the dogs go crazy.*

I chuckled at each note. Some of the resolution failure stories told on
the notes were ones I had experienced myself. Others were just plain
entertaining. I couldn't resist reading every single one.

My favorite:

*If you can figure out how to use this contraption, you can have
it for free!*

Resolutions. We all make them. Most of us don't keep them long.
Some of us have basements or garages filled with items to help us
keep our promises to ourselves or loved ones. Others get tired of
tripping over the contraptions and garb that clutter up our homes...
so they have a huge "resolution sale"!

~Mary Davis

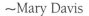

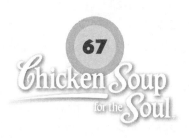

67

Restitution Resolution

I am having an out of money experience.
~Author Unknown

ny fool can pay bills if they have the money. It's paying them when you don't have the money that requires intelligence and resolve.

I've tried a number of different resolutions to solve this problem—all of them time-honored, all of them bad.

First, I tried not paying the bills at all. That didn't work too well. I began to wonder if the power company went out of its way to hire bill adjusters with names like Harlene Hammer and Harvey Fist, or if people with names like that were simply drawn to that sort of work.

Next, I tried gambling. I rigged up a home version of *Wheel of Fortune* so that now, when it's time to pay bills, I can spin for the lucky winners of this month's payments. I've put the mortgage on a few different spaces, but can I help it if their number just doesn't come up?

My husband wanted to make it more rational: Accounts Payable, Accounts Receivable, Accounts Laughable, Accounts Inconceivable.... "I like this," I said. "I'll be Accounts Receivable, you be Accounts Payable. Now write me a check."

"Why?"

"Because I'm broke, and I need to receive some money."

We even went to a financial consultant. Financial Planner, he called himself—though he had less idea than we had about what to "plan" with no money.

"First, you've got to figure out where your money is going," he told us.

Great. If we knew that, we wouldn't need him! Just like when you tell people you've lost your wallet, or your glasses, or your car keys. All helpfulness, they respond, "Well, where'd you last see them?"

Next, the consultant said I should keep track of expenses. But I tried that a few years ago, and it didn't help very much. For months, I carried a notebook around in my purse. I kept meticulous notes: "Tuesday, June 1st: coffee and roll, $1.85; parking meter, $.25; magazine, $2.29; Miscellaneous, $235.00." Somehow I never recorded the details of any purchase larger than ten dollars.

Meanwhile, we keep getting mail from people who wanted to help "invest" our money. I tell them all the same thing: "You've got it," I say, "just as soon as you help us find some."

"Oh no," they all reply. "That's something you'll have to do for yourself. But come to us when you're done." Just like the Little Red Hen. No one's around to help you make ends meet, but as soon as you do, they're there to help you get rid of it. Well, no thanks, I can do that myself.

My real problem, I suspect, is that I'm partial to partial payments. Given a choice of paying $1,000 a year, or $100 a month, I go for the monthly payments every time. "But that costs $200 more a year!" my husband exclaimed. "Why would anyone do that?"

"Maybe," I tell him, "because I have the $200, but if I write a check for a thousand dollars, it will bounce."

Of course, nowadays, nothing need do anything so vulgar as bounce. It just hits bottom and keeps on going, into the black hole of credit card debt.

I was so glad when my mathematician-brother introduced me to the concept of Imaginary numbers. Aha! I thought—now maybe I can balance my checkbook! Only one catch. It seems the banks were all using imaginary numbers, too. Oh well. At least we'll have a lot of high-class company, swimming in the Bankruptcy Pool.

The best suggestion, so far, comes from the history books. I believe it was Abraham Lincoln who used to say "You can pay some of the bills all of the time, and all of the bills some of the time; but you can't pay all of the bills, all of the time." And if it was good enough for Honest Abe, it's good enough for me.

~Judy Epstein

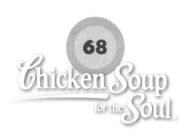

68

Reality TV Resolutions

All television is educational television.
The question is: what is it teaching?
~Nicholas Johnson

It happens like clockwork. I start the beginning of each new year ready for change, stoked for a slimmer, trimmer Al. No, I don't mean hitting the gym—although that would also be a great resolution—but with the promise to give up the reality TV addiction.

Sounds great, huh?

After all, there are so many other issues requiring my attention; and life is too darn short to worry about who wins this year's competition in singing, dancing, cooking, sewing, and surviving in a Third World country, back-stabbing, mind reading, etc.

"This year will be different," I tell myself. "I will focus on getting that promotion at work or fixing up the little things around the house; I will not waste my time lounging on a sofa like a couch potato.... a reality TV junkie."

So I begin my own twelve-step program by just saying "NO." I underscore this watered down cold turkey method by immersing myself in one results-driven project after another. Last year, for example, I built a backyard patio and put in a small water fountain. This year, I've decided to write a book aimed at young adults who want to write.

A week later, my "program" appears to be working. I've seen

nary a reality TV show and I've outlined half the book. Of course, January is a pretty slow month for reality TV. The main ratings titans, i.e., *American Idol* and the dancing competitions, have yet to launch their new seasons. Plus, the media is still reporting on last year's champions—record deals, fashion lines, and various tidbits—which prevent the whole closure thing from hitting us.

Then something happens. It's called February, and sometime during that bitterly cold month, that reality TV juggernaut, *American Idol*, begins traveling city-to-city across the nation holding one bizarre audition after another. That's when I, and many other Americans it would seem, tune in to witness our country's most highly anticipated voting competition. Sure, we want to gauge the best singers before the final twenty-four are announced; but let's face it, we're also intrigued by those auditioning nut cases; those strange creepies who don wild outfits or add unusual elements to their acts; anything to give them the edge on the competition. Yeah, observing these loonies trying to warble their way past the judges proves—once again—riveting.

Also, at that time, I realize that my twelve-step program is flawed. This is largely due to the fact that several steps are missing. Just saying no and filling my life with diversions makes for a good beginning, but what about the remaining tiers, including a support system? My math may be lax, but having two initial strategies does not add up to twelve steps.

After several years, you'd think I would design a better program instead of assuming inner strength would persevere.

So, rather than accepting complete failure, I always latch onto Plan B. That's right; I downsize my reality TV viewing.

After a reality TV inventory, I decide to let a few of the lesser impact shows go (this year, I've settled on *Supernanny* and a few others that don't have that competitive element to their format) and to just enjoy a handful of shows per season. This way, I still get my reality TV fix and yet I notice my housework is more-or-less getting done and I'm able to finish those smaller projects around the house. Writing the young adult book, however, may require more than one season—err, year—which is fine by me. After all, now I have a project I can carry over into next year's resolution period.

In the meantime, I've accepted the realization that I cannot give up *American Idol*. Such a life change will never happen with me. A vicarious participant, I can't help but place myself in the shoes of the contestants, although I know that I'm too old and I do not possess the vocal skills necessary to belt out a Celine Dion tune. But none of that matters to me. The competition of winning this sing-off is simply addictive to me, awakening my competitive—if not irrational—spirit. I somehow believe that by religiously watching this program I am competing.

Truth is, I would be one of those loonies in the auditioning round lambasted by Randy, Simon, and even Paula; my fifteen minutes of fame pared down to mere seconds.

But isn't that the allure of reality TV, to put yourself on that stage with those other competitors?

This is not to say my yearly resolution program has failed. Over the years, I have seen improvement. Gone are the days when I'd record dozens of reality programs at once. Now I have my select few. As for my friends—well, since most of them watch reality TV on a regular basis—they, like me, go into a sort of hibernation during the heavy reality TV season of February to June, re-emerging for the annual A.I. Finale party at someone's home.

I tell myself that someday I will become stronger, that maybe I'll reach a point when I remove reality TV completely from my life. Of course, I will have to tweak my twelve-step program a bit, to make it a bit more complete. But, all things considered, my New Year's resolution track record isn't all that bad. Over the past decade, I've given up smoking and weekly poker nights, so there definitely has been some improvement, some successful resolutions.

Still, my greatest fear is that each season's new crop of reality TV will offer something so totally irresistible that I'll fall off the wagon, erasing the few accomplishments that I have to my credit. Then the next thing I know I'll find myself standing up in front of a bunch of gray-haired strangers in a support group mumbling those twelve horrible words:

"Hi, my name is Al, and I am a reality TV addict."

~Al Serradell

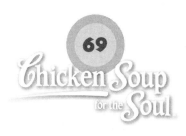

69

Recycling Monster

I love being married. It's so great to find that one special person
you want to annoy for the rest of your life.
~Rita Rudner

Just yesterday I was reminiscing about the good old days. I was remembering how easy and simple life used to be for me and my family. But that was before. Before... recycling. Before... when there were no detailed and lengthy rules and discussions about trash; you just took it out and threw everything in the garbage cans. And all garbage cans looked alike; they were all kind of gray and dented. And, most of the time, the lids didn't really fit. So what changed? Our family resolved to go green and recycle. That challenge turned into the invasion of the Recycling Monster!

Recycling Monster was very cunning and smart. He didn't just come in the front door and plop himself down on the couch. He crept in little by little. And he looked a lot like my husband, Frank. He was gentle and kind and suggested that we, as a family, needed to start a recycling program at home. Our city was initiating its own plan and would help residents wanting to participate in the program by delivering color-coded trash cans — green for garden clippings, blue for paper, plastic and glass, and brown for good old regular trash. How nice. The cans were free, prettier than our old ugly gray cans, and all of the lids fit. So our "going green" adventures began.

The problems started almost immediately. We could all figure out the trash part pretty easily. But then we had to learn what was actually recyclable and what should be considered trash; and who could remember what went with what? Some plastic was considered trash and some was to be recycled. Who knew? It all looked like plastic to me. Some glass went with certain plastics but not with all plastics. Did the lids from the jars stay with the glass or did they go with the metal? Some junk mail was considered trash and some we needed to recycle. I was instructed that if it was printed in red ink we were not to recycle it. Why? Wasn't it all paper? And aluminum foil; don't even ask about the foil. It seems that I was supposed to wash it off before it went into the recycle bin; otherwise it was too sticky and icky to recycle. Imagine, here I was washing my trash before dumping it! Didn't I have better things to do? What had this monster done to my life?

And then things turned ugly. Recycle Monster started picking through the trash, checking up on me. I would put a plastic container in the recycle bin. Recycle Monster would walk by and, not so subtly, he would remove the container and check the number printed on the bottom. We always knew when I had made a mistake because he would proclaim in his best Recycling Monster voice, "Gotcha!"

"What number is on this plastic package?" he would growl. I could tell he was displeased.

"Seven."

"Well, excuse me, but anything with a seven on it is trash. Do not, repeat, DO NOT, put it in with the recyclables. Gotcha!"

To add insult to injury, the city kept changing the rules on us. They would issue new lists of what was and what was not recyclable almost every month. One month the plastic bags from the market were considered trash; the next month they were to be recycled. One month the trays that meat is packaged on were trash; the next month they were to go in the blue can. Recycle Monster was enjoying every minute of this confusion. What happened to the mild-mannered boy from Brooklyn who I married? He couldn't remember where he put his car keys, but he could remember all of the constantly changing recycling rules. They must go in the same part of the male brain as sports scores.

• • •

So how are things today at our house? Not like the good old days, but definitely less tense. Things are not as simple as they were before we resolved to commit to this recycling routine but they are better. Our going green attitude has not been easy for us to maintain, but we are trying. Recycling Monster and I have called a truce. I do the best I can to put everything in its correct bin and the Monster does his best not to let me know when I have made a mistake. If I goof, he just quietly puts the item in the right place... most of the time. Every once in a while a "gotcha" will escape from his lips, but for the most part, he is a reformed monster.

~Barbara LoMonaco

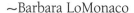

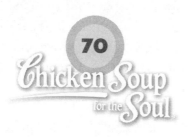

70

Resolving Those Issues

Though no one can go back and make a brand new start,
anyone can start from now and make a brand new ending.
~Author Unknown

Okay, kids, it's that time of year again, when resolutions replace reality in terms of sheer fun to play with. Yes, I know I do this every year, and yes, you can safely assume that some of these are repeats because, yes, my relentless pursuit of perfection is just that—a pursuit. If I actually attained it, I'd be pretty darn hard to live with, now, wouldn't I?

In the spirit of pretending I could actually be a better person someday, here is my list of this year's potential dos, do betters, and do nots. As usual, I reserve the right to add to or delete from this list as the mood strikes.

First, and absolutely most importantly, I resolve to never, ever again ask a woman if she's pregnant unless and until I actually see her giving birth. Not that I've done this twice in the last year or anything.

When I get angry at my children, I will employ the more standard threats of time-outs and groundings, instead of the more personally satisfying threat of getting a real job outside the home.

I will not wait until guests are coming to clean the bathrooms. I say this one every year, but darn it, this is my year! I can feel it!

I will try very, very hard to look at young women with no facial hair and be happy for their youth, instead of silently cursing, "It'll happen to you, sweet thing. Don't you worry, it'll happen to you."

Instead of immaturely jockeying for space when my children climb into our bed in the middle of the night after a bad dream, I will appreciate the precious moments of cuddling that I know will be but a memory soon enough. And I will no longer push my husband off his side so that we have enough room. It'll be more like a gentle nudge.

I will make a concerted effort to put things away after I take them out. This drives my husband nuts, I'm afraid... which makes it all the more difficult to give up! Hahaha.

I will resist the temptation to believe that every headache is a brain tumor, every stomach problem an ulcer, and every memory issue, early-onset Alzheimer's, simply because I might need some attention. And the corollary....

I will start paying attention to myself. When I start thinking that I don't need a shower because the plants didn't die when I walked past, then I will know I'm starting to slip.

I will no longer discourage my son from playing with a certain friend whose mother is younger, thinner, and cuter than I am. It's not as though he can leave me for a better model.

I... will... force... myself to do arts and crafts with my daughter in the mornings before her afternoon pre-K. I can no longer in good conscience tell her that mommy's allergic to paint just because I don't like to clean it up, and I can't expect her to sleep until noon just because I can.

Okay, that's ten. That should do it. I like to work with even numbers. Ooh! Ooh! That brings up another resolution! I resolve to stop rounding our checkbook to the nearest zero. This is another one that drives the husband nuts, but darn it, I've got to give it a shot anyway.

Which of course brings my tally to eleven... an odd number. But that's okay; it's a new me this year, a more flexible me. I'm one step closer to being a better wife and mother, one step closer to perfection, one step closer to... well, being impossible to live with.

Although how that goal differs from reality, I'm not exactly sure.

~Maggie Lamond Simone

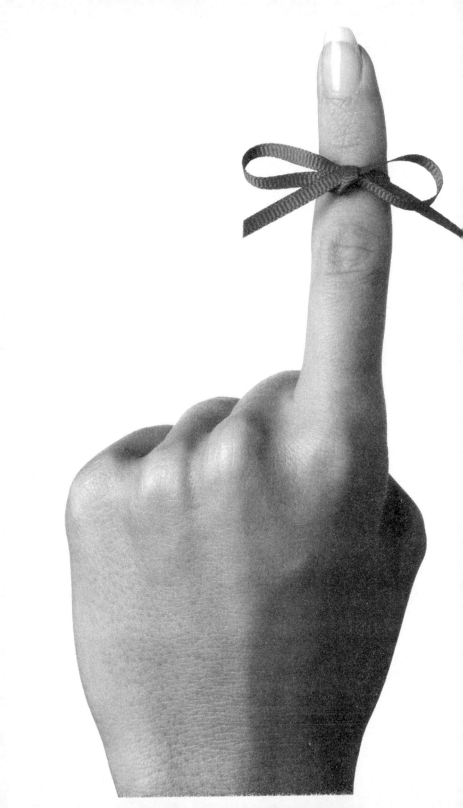

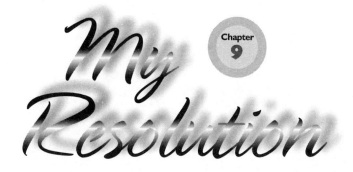

Chapter 9

With You by My Side

A good character is the best tombstone.
Those who loved you and were helped by you will remember you when
forget-me-nots have withered.
Carve your name on hearts, not on marble.

~Charles H. Spurgeon

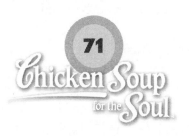

71

A Leap of Faith

A marriage is two people trying to dance a duet
and two solos at the same time.
~Anne Taylor Fleming

"Come and work with me," my husband blurted out one Saturday morning.

"Work with you? Like what, just for today?" I asked.

"No, quit your job and work with me fulltime."

"Are you nuts? Marriage and working together don't mix."

"But I have to let the office girls go. We can't afford the overhead. You can do the work better and faster anyway."

We owned a small business selling tools. The two girls answered the phones, did the invoicing, filing, and all accounting and bookkeeping. We had a shipping guy in the back and one other salesman. I knew things weren't very good, but I didn't think they were that bad.

I already had a fulltime job as a secretary. I liked my boss, my health benefits, vacation time and the perks of a twenty-five-person office that celebrated birthdays and made you feel special. Why would I want to leave all that?

"I don't think working together is a good idea," I said. "I haven't heard of very many marriages that work out when the couple is together 24/7."

"But I need you there."

"That doesn't mean it would be good for us. What about our relationship?"

"We could resolve to make it work."

"Let's think about this," I said, trying to buy some time to get my emotions and thoughts in order. "I'm going upstairs to make the bed."

I almost ran up the steps and into our bedroom. I walked over to the mirror and started brushing my hair. Thoughts barreled one over the other. Was I crazy to even consider this? We'd be in each other's faces with problems and questions and financial issues and phone calls. And what about setting boundaries like going home at a decent hour? I could see us working twelve or fourteen hour days. Would I have to go in early, like he does? I like getting into the office at 9:00 and leaving at 5:00. I set down the hairbrush, walked over to the bed, and yanked up the sheet. Even with the best of intentions and resolutions there's no way this would ever work. I threw the pillows toward the head of the bed, and then pulled the comforter up with such force it flew halfway to the top. He's got some nerve to ask me to do such a thing.

The rest of the day neither one of us broached the subject. But on Sunday night he brought it up again. "So, did you think about it?"

"I did. And I still don't like the idea."

The next morning I went into work and, over a cup of coffee, told a few close girlfriends about my dilemma. "You're crazy. If I ever worked with my husband, I'd kill him," said one. "Don't do it. It'll be the death of your marriage," said another. "I can't get through a weekend without having some kind of argument with my spouse," said the receptionist when she came in and filled her cup. "I like it just fine when we both go our separate ways on Monday."

They were right. There were pitfalls in the plan. Financially it made sense, but I couldn't shake the feeling that our marriage would be in trouble.

"Honey," I said when we both were home that night, "I've given it a lot of thought."

"And?"

"I'm worried you'll holler at me when things go wrong, and I'll get all over your case about things you don't do right."

"Then let's make a division of labor. You handle all the office stuff, and I'll handle the sales and shipping."

"I make the decisions in the front?"

"Yup, and I'll do all the work in the back."

"That might be good..." I whispered, but something nagged at me.

"What are you thinking?" my husband said.

"That our marriage is more important than work. Our relationship comes first."

"I totally agree. I'll tell you what. If it doesn't work out, you can quit."

"I can quit?"

"Resolve to give it six months. If you don't like it, leave."

My mind starting spinning. I wondered if they'd take me back at my old job if I left. If we let the two office girls go, and I did the work for six months, who would do it if I quit? Somehow, though, just the thought of being able to get out if I wanted to felt good.

"Well, that's something to consider. But it's not about the work. It's about us. If it isn't working for our marriage, then I'll leave because our relationship is the most important thing."

"Deal."

"For real?" I questioned.

"For real. At six months, and every six months after that if you stay, we'll sit down and talk. We'll discuss what's working, and what isn't. How you like the hours, the job itself, and how you like working with me. And me with you."

"You may think I'm a pain in the butt to work with."

"Maybe. We'll both have an out. Okay?"

"Okay."

The next Monday he gave the girls their two-week notice and I gave mine. My boss begged and pleaded for me to stay, but how could he argue against my reason for leaving?

With strong resolve, but some trepidation, I began my new job. Some of the work I was used to. Over the years I had come in on various weekends with my husband and cleaned up things that needed to be done. What I wasn't used to was how my husband maintained his office. I was a neat freak. He wasn't. I liked to arrive and leave at a reasonable time. He always had something more to do.

So I started driving myself in every morning instead of coming in together. That extra hour or two at home made a huge difference in my mental attitude. And I left at 5:00 to make dinner a few times a week. We negotiated a schedule of eating out or picking something up the other nights.

And his messy desk versus my clean one? Well, that came to a head right away.

"Can you help me find a file? It's here in my office somewhere," my husband called out one day.

"It's a black hole in there," I called back from my chair. "Everything that goes into that place gets sucked in and never comes out."

"You're better at finding things than I am. Can you help me?"

"Okay," I responded, and walked into his office. "But if I find what you're looking for, you owe me a dollar."

Years later, those dollars multiplied to hundreds, but who's counting? And that escape clause? There were times I wrote in huge, big, black letters "I QUIT" on a white sheet of paper and flashed it at him from his office doorway. We smiled, then laughed, and got over what irked us at the time.

Every six months we talk about our relationship. It was rocky at first, that's for sure, but fifteen years later, we still work together, side by side. I'm really glad I took that leap of faith. Now, I wouldn't have it any other way.

~B.J. Taylor

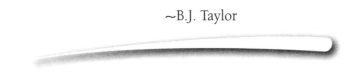

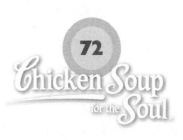

72

It Helps to Have a Friend

A true friend reaches for your hand and touches your heart.
~Author Unknown

"Mm, good coffee," said my next door neighbor, Virginia, pushing aside the folded laundry on my couch. "What kind? And what'd you do to your finger?"

"You noticed," I said gingerly holding my cup between my thumb and third finger. "Chocolate Raspberry and I bit my nail and cuticle back too far."

"You're a nail biter?" she asked, dismissing the name of my favorite flavored coffee.

"Yeah," I admitted. "It's my life-long, childhood habit."

"When do you do it?" she asked, leaning over the coffee table and eyeballing me.

I straightened a little. "When do I do what? Make flavored coffee? Only when you come over. Bill doesn't like it. He says it is women's coffee."

"Your nails, silly," she said, laughing. "When do you bite your nails?"

I shrugged. "How do I know? All the time, I guess. If I don't bite them, I pick them off. It really only hurts when I get them too short or get an infection."

Virginia gasped. "You got an infection from biting your nails?"

"Uh-huh," I said, "It happens when my wounded little fingers go swimming in dirty dishwater." I tried to be nonchalant, but Virginia wouldn't turn loose.

"I'll help you quit," she volunteered.

"It's a lost cause," I countered. "I've tried to quit all my life. When I was a little girl my aunt offered me five dollars to quit, but I couldn't."

"Well, for the next two weeks I'm going to come over every morning and give you a manicure," she announced. "Together we're going to kick your habit!"

"Every morning?" I said in disbelief. "What do you think you're going to manicure, the ends of my fingers?"

"You'll see," she said. "I won't stay long, just long enough to do your nails."

The next morning, Virginia was at my kitchen door with a tray full of manicuring equipment. The sun streamed in the breakfast nook window as she spread my hands out flat on the table. She surveyed the damage and set right to work.

"First we have to file off the rough places and trim the snags," she said.

There wasn't much to file but she filed and filed. Then she gently pushed back my cuticles and trimmed off snags.

"Ow!" I said when she pushed on a tender spot. My fingers weren't overjoyed with the attention, but I was intrigued that she would spend so much time on such awful-looking hands. Finally she opened a small bottle of clear nail polish and carefully polished each stub as if it were a magnificently long nail.

"There!" she said triumphantly. "See you tomorrow." She quickly loaded up her tray and left.

I sat there a long time looking at my shiny stubs. No one had ever spent that much time caring for them before, especially not me.

That afternoon I attacked a long put-off project. I spread fabric on the floor and took out the pattern for my new dress. As I worked to place the pattern pieces just right before cutting, I felt my bottom teeth rub against a fingernail. I quickly separated the two. Within a minute I felt it again.

"I'll ruin the polish," I wailed.

By the third time, I realized my hand had a mind of its own, bypassing my brain.

The next morning Virginia came again. She took a cotton ball and some polish remover and took off yesterday's polish. The nicks smarted, but I didn't complain. Again she filed and filed, pushed back cuticles, painted stubs, and was gone.

Later in the day, when I was working on my grocery list, I discovered my left hand in my mouth. I quickly retrieved it and sat on it while I completed the list.

Every day for a week Virginia came over and did a complete manicure. She filed so much I feared my nails would never grow, but they looked and felt so much better because the surrounding tissue was no longer inflamed.

Gradually, as I became aware of where my hands were, I could keep them in my lap or wherever else my brain directed them. No longer did they subconsciously go to my mouth. My nails had become my focal point because Virginia cared about them. And I was learning to care, too.

At the end of two weeks there was a smooth band of white around the tip of each nail.

"We're going to switch to twice a week now," Virginia said. She laughed. "I'll have to see if I can break my new habit of Chocolate Raspberry coffee."

The last time Virginia came to do my nails, she brought a bottle of shocking pink polish. She polished and I "oohed and ahhed" as I displayed a set of long, polished nails. Then she pronounced me "graduated."

So was I no longer tempted by a crunchy nail treat? Hardly! I found that every three or four months I had to reinforce my decision and new habit. Virginia suggested that I temporarily cover the evidence of any fingernail attack with a press-on nail, refocus on where my hands were, and start manicuring again.

I found myself frequently whispering, "Thank you, Lord, for a friend who cared enough to help me break my nail-biting habit." Otherwise, I might never have tried.

~Pauline Youd

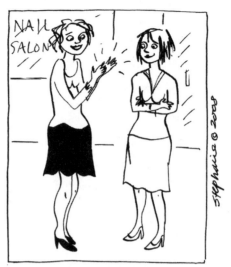

"The only way I could stop
biting my nails was to get
a manicure. I can't bring
myself to ruin anything
so expensive!"

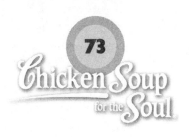

Keeping My Head Above Water

A friend accepts us as we are yet helps us to be what we should.
~Author Unknown

"How far can I go?" I often wondered, as I swam at my health club. I knew I had stamina and strength to swim an hour's worth of laps, but I had never tested "other waters."

So when my friend Sue invited me to visit her at the lake house, I eagerly accepted. "The lake stretches for miles," she told me. I had always admired my triathlete friends who churned their way across large bodies of water. I knew I would feel so strong and proud if I could swim across a real lake.

"How do I get in?" I asked, as Sue and I stood on the dock. The lake yawned, smooth, empty and inviting. There were no ropes, no motorboats, no boundaries of any kind.

"Jump," Sue said, surprised by my question.

"And how do I get out?"

"Hoist yourself up, or wade out. Haven't you ever been in a lake?"

As a child, I had one lake experience. We drove for several hours to reach a lake with a real sand beach. Before we could rush down to the water, my mother warned: "Don't go beyond the ropes." The ropes surrounded a small square of water, not much larger than our backyard. Beyond the ropes beckoned rafts, docks and sailboats. I had watched enviously as an Irish Setter paddled out exuberantly past the confines.

Now, I was finally going "beyond the ropes." I looked at the greenish-brown water. I was used to swimming in a crowded pool and easing in with a ladder. I was not used to mud bottoms, floating twigs and water spiders.

I closed my eyes and jumped in. After the initial bite of coolness, I began a crawl stroke. What luxury, not thinking about keeping within the lanes, not having any sides to bump into, any people to watch out for. I stretched my body and enjoyed the sound of my legs kicking.

I glanced back and could not see the dock; I looked ahead and could not yet see the opposite shore. Suddenly I realized I was alone in deep water. There were rules about being alone in deep water: never do it. My stomach clenched; I felt panic. What if I cramped? What if I couldn't make it back to the dock? What if I had gone too far?

I assured myself that I swam an hour every day and this day need not be different. I had also taken a special "drownproofing" class and knew how to stay afloat for hours. I was ready. I could do this.

But voices in my head chanted: "It's too far, you're too weak." I accidentally breathed in water and choked. Shaken, I backstroked towards shore.

"You're just not used to the freedom," Sue told me.

"You can do this," I said every morning as I got into the lake. My mother had said these words to me when I first took swimming lessons. Those very words inspired me to swallow my panic, along with a lot of water, and somehow pass my Minnow test.

Now I was far beyond Minnow. Still, as I got into deeper water, my own invisible boundaries rushed in. I always turned back before I'd gotten halfway.

On my last day, I swam quickly, figuring if I kept moving I wouldn't be afraid.

As I moved into the center of the lake, the water temperature grew colder and the voices in my head grew louder: "It's too deep, you'll drown." The edges of land blurred. "You are in over your head." My stomach cramped. My legs felt heavy, my arms shaky. I can do this, I thought, trying to stave off panic. I continued swimming until my breath was ragged and my teeth were fidgety with cold. I was closer to the far shore than I'd been all week when I had to turn back.

Several days later, I was back in the health club pool, telling my lane mate, a seasoned triathlete, about my lake fiasco. He snapped his swim cap over his buzz cut and straightened his goggles. "I swam from Alcatraz to San Francisco," he said. "My girlfriend rowed beside me."

I looked at him in astonishment. A tough, macho guy like him with a safety net! I never thought of asking someone to go with me: I assumed I had to conquer deep water alone.

I resolve to go back to the lake next year. But first, I'm going to ask Sue how she feels about rowing across the lake. Maybe just knowing she is there will give me the courage to go the distance.

~Deborah Shouse

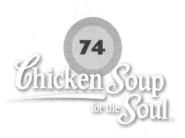

The Quest

An adventure is only an inconvenience rightly considered.
An inconvenience is only an adventure wrongly considered.
~G.K. Chesterton

had heard about the Florida International University writing class from my girlfriend, Becky. "It's one day a week. We can handle that. I know it's a long way, but if you're willing to drive, I'll go."

Becky is not only my oldest friend, but she is also a fearless, middle-aged immigration attorney with a kind heart and a bad sense of direction. Sometimes I tell her it's because of her Puerto Rican heritage, just to irk her. But the truth is, my sense of direction is much worse than hers. Between the two of us we can't find our way out of Bloomingdale's. But I felt that I needed her courage to lead me.

"I'll do it." As I said the words I felt the adrenaline rush. More than anything else, I wanted to go to this class, but fear was taking over now and I knew I couldn't let it.

When I was growing up, I didn't have the opportunity to go to college. My mother had become ill when I was fourteen, and I took various part-time jobs to help out financially. I focused on trying to earn a living, not studying. In high school, I never opened a book. I squeaked by and was reminded regularly by the nuns at my high school that I didn't have a shot of getting into college. Maybe I wasn't smart enough? It didn't bother me. I knew I'd survive. I'd heard that a starting salary for lawyers back then was about $12,000. I knew I could make at least that if I joined an airline. I did; I've never been sorry. I've had the kind of life most people only dream about.

But as I got dangerously close to turning fifty, things began to look different. Middle age allows you see things that you didn't see before. You wonder what would have happened if.... What if I had gone to college? Is it too late?

I'd been pleading with Becky to take a writing class with me for over a year; now she was breaking down and agreeing to go. This was my chance to find out.

On the two-hour ride to Florida International University (traffic in Miami is horrible) we realized that it was the last day of registration. We wondered if it was too late to get into the class. Becky and I wandered around the campus in the heat, asking everyone we could for directions to the Admissions Office. There, we joined a long line. An hour later, a striking young Haitian woman, who never once smiled, shoved a form at us and told us to fill it out and bring it back. Becky and I found seats on a wooden bench and studied the form. When we got to "education," Becky filled in Immigration Attorney; I left mine blank. We got back in the line, which now extended out the door and around the building, and waited.

Standing in line, I felt anxious, afraid that when it was my turn the woman behind the desk would ask me if I had been to college. What would I say? No, but it's never too late. I've had a successful life, anyway. I wasn't bright enough? How trite. I nervously fumbled with my form, bending the sides of the paper. The woman behind the desk glared at Becky's paperwork and then asked what level of education had she completed?

My hands shook. I knew she was going to ask me the same question.

Becky answered that she was an immigration attorney. The woman grimaced. "Well then, you spelled street wrong." What she really meant was: "So, for an educated woman, you can't spell?"

Suddenly, I had a vision of Becky reaching down, pulling a knife from her Manolo Blahnik heels, placing it between her teeth, while at the same time, singing the "When You're a Jet" theme song from *West Side Story*, as she lunged at the woman.

"Well, I didn't go to college and I got that one right," I said trying to ease the tension.

The woman was not amused by our antics; she assigned us a PIN number, and pointed to the computers across the room, on the far side of the wall. "Go register." This time I detected a faint smile. She thinks we're computer illiterate. She's right.

I glared at the computers and sighed deeply. The lines were longer now than before; we waited for another hour. Becky took the first computer when it became available. And when the next one came up, I grabbed it. I noticed that my computer was lower to the ground than the others were. From this angle, my fingers had trouble reaching the keys, so I placed my paperwork on the floor next to me, and got on my hands and knees. The thought that the computer had been designed for the physically challenged never occurred to me. I played with the keys trying to locate my ID number and grew more frustrated. What was an ID number, anyway? The screen flashed insufficient information.

I guess the student standing behind me felt sorry for me because she leaned over to help, but in order to reach the keyboard she also had to get on her hands and knees. With a few strokes, she was able to log on and find the class that I was looking for.

The next thing I knew, someone tripped over her, and then another person fell, and then another, like a row of dominoes, all going down at once. I apologized to everyone around me and out of sheer embarrassment, focused on the screen which now blinked. Class full. Class full. Class full.

As Becky and I drove home from FIU, she explained how much we'd accomplished. "We found the school, and we got a PIN. Next time, we'll be ready. At least, now we know the system."

It's funny how two people can see different sides of the same story. She saw it as a total success; I saw it as a dismal failure. Maybe, I wasn't ready for the big time yet. Maybe college was more than I could handle? Maybe, I'm a health hazard to the other students and faculty?

The next day I saw an ad for the Institute for Retired Professionals. IRP is a division of the University of Miami, and its purpose is to continue education for those over fifty. The flyer read: "Make creative writing a part of your life. Learn to tell your story."

I called Becky. "Guess what? I've found another writing course. This one is perfect for us."

"Oh God, not again," she said. "What time does the class start?"

~Joyce Newman Scott

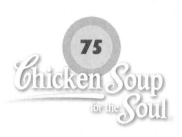

Winning the Battle of the Bulge

A diet is the penalty we pay for exceeding the feed limit.
~Author Unknown

"This New Year's resolution makes me feel like we're enlisting in WWII," Ed remarked as we sat in the car waiting for our noon meeting and our second tour of duty with a structured weight loss program.

"Honey, it's not like we're facing a firing squad," I said, although I couldn't help but be amused by his flair for the dramatic.

"Maybe after a few weight loss meetings we'll get back into the swing of dieting," I said, attempting to look at the bright side of our on-going Battle of the Bulge. Ed didn't reply. He heaved a weary sigh thinking of the challenge that lay ahead for us.

I knew where Ed was coming from. Losing weight is a struggle I've faced since I was a teenager. Counting calories and watching my daily intake had become second nature to me by the time I was in my early twenties.

On the flip side, my husband, Ed, didn't start having a weight problem until he reached his mid-forties. Active and naturally slender, he never had to concern himself with the caloric difference between a pound of peanut butter fudge and a pound of celery sticks. In some ways, I feel worse for him than I do for myself. Along with being familiar with caloric values, I altered my eating habits when I was young, while Ed had to change deep-rooted habits with little knowledge of how to make wise food choices.

When we were still living in Seattle, Ed lost fifty-six pounds and I lost eighteen while attending regular weight loss meetings. Our weight didn't just disappear; we fought with great determination to re-shape our bodies and improve our overall health. What a rewarding feeling to know we had faced the enemy and won! We'd mastered the Battle of the Bulge, and amazingly we'd done it by following a program that didn't include ice cream as one of the major food groups.

We earned our Good Conduct medals during our WWI tour, but not without hard battles. At the first meeting, our fellow comrades let us know that munching on macadamia nuts during the meeting was not acceptable, and moreover, not offering to share was behavior unbecoming to the weight loss club.

A few weeks later, forgetting the earlier skirmish over the macadamia incident, Ed stood up after a particularly rousing weight loss meeting, and asked, "How about we all go for Mexican food after the meeting?" Everyone in the room joined us.

The following week the Drill Sergeant, AKA the red-faced weight loss instructor, took us aside and pointed out the potential physical dangers of mentioning any kind of forbidden food in a room full of club members who aren't related to Twiggy. She was clearly very perturbed with us.

Soon after losing the weight in Seattle, our lives took a turn, and we made a major move to the Southwest. With a new job and a new home in the Land of Enchantment, success was felt on all fronts, except for one very important one... the scales. Time and our weight had marched on, and the scales said we were in a downward spiral to defeat.

We rationalized that the disruption of the move was the reason for our expanding girth. But the truth is we had grazed our way 1,900 miles south, by treating ourselves at some of the most decadent ice cream shops America had to offer.

So, after months of putting off the inevitable, we had no choice but to re-enlist for WWII. We are much wiser now that we've re-upped for a second tour of duty, and we want to do everything just right.

Our desire to reduce during this second tour has prompted us to seek out and experiment with new and alternative foods. Our kitchen table is a war planning zone for charting the calories we've eaten and those we've yet to consume. Our goals in meeting the enemy head-on include searches for recipes promising low fat, low sugar and low calories.

We've been studying our weight loss books. I've pulled out my low everything recipes and removed from the refrigerator and cupboards the foods that could be toxic to the mission. We've enlisted our dachshund, Leon, to join the program. I've even removed the clothes hangers from the treadmill so it's ready to go into action 24/7.

We feel WWII and the Battle of the Bulge can be won again. The pounds are slowly melting from our bodies, and morale among the troops seems to be sustaining itself. But will our spirits remain high with Ed and me celebrating our successes after the meetings by rushing out to dine on Mexican food?

Losing weight is a treacherous lifelong war; some days we limp into battle and other days we march to victory. However, every day we're thankful for New Year's resolutions that will keep us from being drafted to serve in WWIII.

~Cynthia Briggs

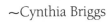

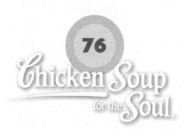

76

Fear and Cheer

*The way you overcome shyness is to become so wrapped up in something
that you forget to be afraid.*
~Lady Bird Johnson

made my resolution at my daughter's National
Cheerleading Competition in Disney World. It was a surprising place for me to make a resolution, given Disney,
cheerleading, and me are an unlikely combination. I am always
more concerned with finding a yoga class and a pretty place to run.
In contrast, my daughter had been eagerly anticipating this trip for
months — training, stretching, and tumbling with the discipline of
an Olympian. "And the rides Mom, now that will be great!"

Great wasn't the first word that came to mind when I thought
about roller coasters in the dark and elevators crashing from the
sky. But it was that kid-like sparkle in her brown eyes which was
the first glimmer of my resolution. I'd always been terrified of scary
rides — safely watching, holding my children's melting ice cream as
they danced in the sky high above. Their laughter and excitement
was a joy to watch, but sharing it would be even better. So as my
daughter hoped to return with a national award, I wanted to return
having championed my fear. She was training to do flips in the air
and I was preparing to fly — holding on for dear life.

All cheerleaders had to be accompanied by a parent chaperone,
and compared to my husband, I'm a pom-pom professional. We
attended numerous meetings with coaches where we were handed

lists, competition schedules, bus schedules, lodging specifics, and rule sheets as we prepared for the launch of two hundred cheerleaders. I'd do my best to be a good cheerleading mom but I also knew I was going to lead a silent cheer for myself that wasn't written on any of the handouts.

I tried to be organized for our adventure, buying my Disney ticket on-line. Unfortunately I proudly purchased a three-day pass to Disneyland in California instead of Disney World in Florida. The smiley woman at guest relations shook her head, apologized and politely handed it back to me. "Y'all will just have to buy a new $250 pass." And then... "All righty, I'll give you a complimentary ticket, but shush now and just keep yourselves movin'." Her small gesture was like a fortune cookie message, "Resolutions can cost nothing, but be worth everything." She suddenly looked enchanting and the Magic Kingdom—just magical.

We spent the weekend in a "clump"—four daughters and four mothers, busing it between competitions. My daughter lives her fourteen-year-old life in a clump, a group project with her friends that is devoted to growing up all too quickly. In contrast I have dear friends but have always appreciated my solitude. Group travel isn't usually my chosen form of transportation. So along with roller coasters and elevators that drop from the sky, I was confronting my shyness in a group of moms, among an even larger group of tourists, bumping elbows, all searching for the electrifying thrill of Disney.

Since it was a freezing weekend in Orlando, I did have to purchase two pairs of Mickey socks to wear with my sandals, which got a few looks from my daughter. But she often finds me embarrassing these days; Mickey socks are the least of it.

But the true warmth came from spending time with the other mothers. Quickly, we stopped talking about the weather, and began sharing our lives, loves, losses, heartaches and laughter. They were patient with me, as I tend to ask curious questions both in and out of my psychotherapy office. My mother always reminds me that at age four I asked a divorced neighbor, "Exactly what didn't you like about your first husband?" Trailing behind four adolescent jabbering girls with large red and blue bows in their hair was contagious. We mothers began to wonder if we'd soon be texting each other, sipping from the same straw and borrowing clothes.

Given that the girls spend much of their lives "getting ready," we all found ourselves stumbling towards our toothbrushes at 5:30 A.M.—preparing for the 7:00 bus launch, with the coach refrain in our head, "DON'T EVER, EVER BE LATE!" With the end of the competition, the girls made us all proud. But for me, my biggest challenge was just beginning. We all "clumped" together to plan our afternoon rides. I found myself saying, "You know I could always sit with a cup of tea and my book." My new friends laughed, letting me know there would be no back door at Disney.

I had already decided that I would need a way to manage my anxiety. I began to think of those moments in yoga class when the soft voice of my teacher guides us through a meditation. I find that place inside where for a moment the world is truly peaceful. I asked my daughter if she'd sit next to me on the elevator ride that drops from the sky. How many nights had she come running in, in the dark, whispering, "Mommy, I'm scared." And now it is my turn to rely on my grown-up daughter. We buckled up laughing and screaming before the ride even began. I tried to breathe in and out and find that yoga place, depending on both myself and my small community to keep me safe. And suddenly WHOOOOSH! We were dropping, shrieking and holding each other tight.

The exhilaration left me tearful and with that childlike feeling of, "Again Mommy, again."

Of course, we did celebrate with another time high in the sky. But the true celebration was getting on board with some dear friends and "clumping it." I learned to rely on strangers who had become friends, reminding me that group travel provides a smoother ride in this wild and spinning world. One resolution has led me to another, which is to risk leaning on others more, because it gives us all the chance to fly. And that is something we can cheer for.

~Priscilla Dann-Courtney

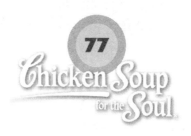

77

"You Didn't Quit, Mommy, So Neither Did I"

Don't worry that children never listen to you;
worry that they are always watching you.
~Robert Fulghum

I truly thought that I might die that day. Had I not seen three bears and a few wolves over the last couple of days near the road, I might have just laid down and called it quits. What in the world was I thinking, dragging my bike up to Yellowstone and thinking I could ride from West Yellowstone to Old Faithful—in the snow, no less! A year ago I would never have believed it.

I don't know what made me decide to change my life. One day in March, I just woke up tired of being fat. I was tired of feeling like my weight defined my whole existence. I wanted to play with my children and to be the kind of mother of whom they could be proud. I convinced my husband that our family could stand to get a little healthier and just like that it began.

I threw myself into discovering better ways to eat. I got all of the sugar and junk food out of the house and replaced it with fresh fruits and vegetables. For the first time in my life, I started to exercise every day. At first it was absolute torture. I kept the phone right by me, just in case I had a heart attack on my stationary bike. I told everyone I knew that I was getting healthy—my pride ensuring that because everyone would be watching, I would try harder. Amazingly, just like it is supposed to, the weight started to come off.

The change spread through my whole family. My husband, who hadn't cycled in years, bought a new road bike and soon convinced me to join him. By June, he had signed me up to do a twenty-two mile charity ride with him. I was scared to death, but I ended up having a fantastic time. It felt so empowering to be in good enough shape to not only finish the ride, but to finish before more than half of the people riding.

Soon I was getting up to ride my bike early every morning. On Saturdays, my husband and I would get a babysitter and ride for a couple of hours. Imagine that! The girl who hated walking a quarter of a mile to school was trading date night at the IHOP for hours on a bike.

By August, I was sixty pounds lighter and in better shape than I had ever been. I coached my daughter's soccer team and ran around doing drills with them. They got winded before I did. I could tell that my daughter was proud of me, and that was inspiration to keep going. Later that month, I completed a sixty-eight mile ride in a little less than five hours total time. Completing that ride was a dream come true and I thought that I could now do anything. Then came Yellowstone....

Had everything gone perfectly, it wouldn't have been so bad. However, besides the weather, I wasn't feeling well and had not eaten properly for such an effort. We had planned this trip for more than two months, though, and I wasn't about to give up so easily. The first few miles were beautiful. Ten miles in, I started sucking wind. Fifteen miles and my legs felt like they were made of lead. By twenty miles, my lungs were burning and I felt like there was nothing left in the tank.

That's when I turned around and saw my three children cheering me on in the van behind me. I knew then that I couldn't quit. I tell my children all the time that just because something is hard doesn't mean that you stop doing it. I had to live what I'd been preaching. That thought and a lot of prayer got me up that mountain and to the end of the ride. It took everything I had and then some, but I made it.

The importance of that ride was apparent after only a week. My eight-year-old daughter Emalee wanted to ride in a twelve mile breast cancer awareness ride. We told her it would not be easy, but we thought that she could do it. That day was cold as well. She was the youngest rider and I was already proud of her for even trying. About four miles into the ride, she started feeling the cold. The chill was making her muscles cramp a little and she began to struggle. By six miles, she had tears running down her face.

It broke my heart to see her suffering like that. I told her that she didn't have to finish, that we could stop and call someone to pick us up. She said that she wouldn't quit. I told her how I had wanted to quit the week before, but that prayer and perseverance had gotten me to the end and I knew that she could do it too.

I don't remember much more of that ride—I was too busy praying for my little girl and trying to keep her safe and inspired. The look on her face as she pulled into the finish was priceless. She threw her arms around me and said "You didn't quit, Mommy, so neither did I." Everything I'd been through for the last seven months was worth it for that one moment when I realized that my daughter wanted to be like me, and for once, that was okay!

~Kimberlee Garrett

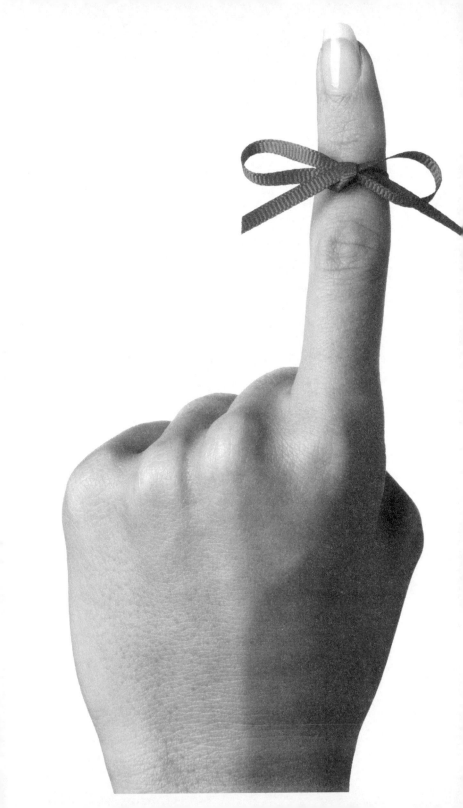

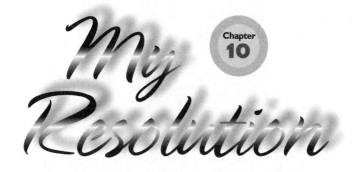

Dreams Do Come True

To change one's life: Start immediately.
Do it flamboyantly. No exceptions.

~William James

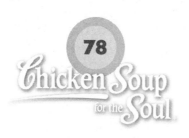

78

Resolving Life

We will open the book. Its pages are blank.
We are going to put words on them ourselves.
The book is called Opportunity and its first chapter is New Year's Day.
~Edith Lovejoy Pierce

My husband and I sit quietly in our family room. The TV is on and we are watching the celebration in Time Square. I am so very tired, but I am trying very hard to stay awake. My eyes want to close but something within my soul drives me to reach the midnight hour. I want to say goodbye to the year 1999 and welcome in the year 2000. Slowly the ball starts to descend and a new year has been established.

Time to make my New Year's resolutions. Always in my life, resolutions never made it to February; the year 2000 was going to be different.

My 1999 calendar was marked with doctor appointments, hospital visits, surgeries and chemotherapies. My 2000 calendar looked much the same; I still had more doctor appointments than social events. All of this happened because of the demon breast cancer.

My resolution for the year 2000 was to LIVE; not just existing as an earthly being, but truly living life. This resolve would be my hardest, but I told myself on that last day of December, 1999, I would be a cancer survivor.

Much like the rest of the world I had also made resolutions to get more exercise, eat healthful meals, and live a better life. Those resolutions were made only to be broken. But I knew on that quiet New Year's Eve that I would live out my resolutions not just for the coming year, but for many years to come.

I resolved to myself that my name would be among the names of other cancer survivors. My health would be restored and never again would I take life for granted. My approach would be to live each day with a positive attitude. I would laugh at life and enjoy every moment. Nothing would stop me from being a wife and mother. My parents would be proud of my accomplishments and my sisters would be pleased to call me Sis. No longer would I be upset over spilled milk, for it was only spilled milk. My eyes would enjoy the beauty that God created and yes, I would take time to smell the roses. My heart would pour out love and my hands would be instruments to help other women living with breast cancer.

I would have courage to take a step in faith, and not just dream, but live those dreams.

I knew that I had some very difficult resolutions before me in the year 2000, but I knew with the love of family and friends I would persevere. There were days when I found myself struggling, but I would remind myself of that quiet day when I chose to become a breast cancer survivor.

Nine years have come and gone. As the ball descends and a new year is born I smile to myself and realize that I am still living those resolutions that were made nine years ago on a quiet wintry night. I am a breast cancer survivor!

~Karen Theis

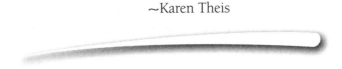

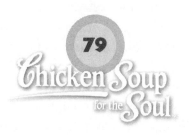

Too Dumb

> *Become a possibilitarian. No matter how dark things seem to be*
> *or actually are, raise your sights and see possibilities—*
> *always see them, for they're always there.*
> ~Norman Vincent Peale

I hear footsteps coming around the darkened corner of book laden aisles. I rush to re-shelve a hardcover book; it slips from my sweaty palm to collide with the concrete floor. Standing rigid, I breathe quietly, praying to be invisible. My prayer answered, the disinterested interloper strolls past. A hasty glance over my shoulder, I jump back inside the cover.

I, a high school drop-out, am standing inside a university bookstore. Walking home every day, after eight hours of serving oily tacos, I have gazed into this window of heaven. But somehow on this day, I find myself standing inside the door; inhaling the delicious scent of ink swirling about, hearing the hushed murmur of solemn voices.

A full five minutes pass and no one orders me outside. I step over to the nearest bookshelf. *Introduction to Accounting.* I groan. Numbers and I are like little boys and baths. I move to another shelf, smile as I skim sideways titles.

Then, the unbelievable. A book reaches out and refuses to allow me to pass. I stand there, eyes wide open. Loneliness, the low paying job, my self-assigned place in the world, all evaporate. I gathered my courage, scrutinize the room. And reach out my hand, pick up the heavy maroon tome and hold it against me.

Too Dumb : Dreams Do Come True   277

No clerk comes running over to remove it from me. The ink stinks delightfully. I feel the smooth shiny surface and smile at the rich color. I hear the occasional ring of the entrance bell as customers come and go. Holding the heavy text in my left hand, I crack open the stiff jacket with my right hand. *Introduction to Law*. Scanning the title page, I eagerly flip pages, past the introduction, past the....

"Can I help you, ma'am?" I look up to see a pony-tailed student, wearing an employee sign and a wide grin.

I groan. Not only the reminder I am no longer "miss," but my good fortune has ended. I will now be asked to leave. Well, five minutes in heaven is better than....

"That book's not too bad," she runs her finger down the deep red spine of the book I am clutching. I sadly replace the coveted volume, and pull my thin purse strap onto my shoulder.

"Just looking—I'll leave." I stare at the floor; scuff my worn shoe against the shelf. The girl looks at me inquisitively. "You can buy that book used, you know. I just finished that class... learned a lot." Her smile is as friendly as can be. Friendly to me.

"Huh?" I frown at her in disbelief. Me? Take a law class? I'm too dumb for that. "Yeah right, me take a law class? I don't think so." I turn away with a pink face. Wishing I had just gone straight home like always. I don't mind being asked to leave the bookstore, but don't make fun of me like this. Suggesting I take a class like law. Which everyone knows is for smart people.

"Well, you should check it out. I passed." With that the cheerful girl leaves, snapping her bubble gum. And snapping at the balloon of self-denigration I carried with myself in those days.

Didn't this girl know I was a high school drop-out? (I had used that excuse to avoid many challenges). A single parent, a series of low paying jobs; I had labeled myself LOSER in capital letters.

I watch this young lady saunter away, she with the law class under her belt. And I start to wonder "why?" Why am I still the loser? My son is in high school now. He loves me and while we are poor, we have a good life. I have a nice apartment; walk with friends in the evening. Could it be that it is time to dump the "loser" label?

•••

I took the Introduction to Law class. I got a 99%. I enrolled in the paralegal program, sailed through those classes, receiving straight As except for one B+. Working as a paralegal increased my income four-fold and I went on to earn a bachelor's degree. As a college graduate with two degrees, the "loser" label no longer fits.

May I suggest as the new year approaches, you slip into a college bookstore. Walk the aisles until a book reaches out for you. Does your pulse jump a little when you hold it? Sign up for that class; don't wait for a bubble-gum-chewing chick to encourage you. She might be two aisles over. If you carry a "Too Dumb" label, you might decide to leave it behind you. You will not miss it, I promise.

~HJ Eggers

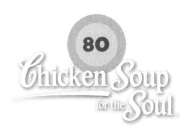

The Life List

Kids spell love T-I-M-E.
~John Crudele

I am not a big fan of resolutions. To me, they seem more like opportunities for failure. Sure, there are those who stick to their guns to lose weight, exercise, or quit smoking. But my resolution is more of a "realization" than a "resolution."

On any typical day, my hectic schedule is fairly routine. I work full-time, come home, exercise (not a resolution—just a healthy choice), and frantically try to accomplish the never-ending household chores between driving my daughter to dance class, school functions, social gatherings and the like. Elizabeth is sixteen, not quite driving on her own, and extremely active. I keep lists and reminders of everything. Our family calendar is frequently updated and you will often find Post-it notes on the kitchen counter as additional reminders. There is little room for spontaneity.

My realization came one evening when Elizabeth asked if I would like to see pictures from her pool party. I believe my response was something like, "I need to finish up the dishes and fold laundry. I'll look at them after that, if it doesn't get too late. Or, I'll look at them tomorrow." I may have even written myself a reminder.

Later, I realized that what should have waited for tomorrow were the dishes and laundry. I was frittering away precious time with Elizabeth. All too soon she would be off to college and on her own. If I'm lucky, there will be occasional weekend visits. (More laundry!)

So what would happen if the sink contained some dirty dishes while Elizabeth and I caught a movie or had a facial? Would the world end if the hamper was full but Elizabeth and I were too busy shopping and going out to eat to care? I was definitely going to make an effort to change my somewhat rigid ways, add some of that spontaneity to our lives, and spend as much time as possible with my daughter right now while I had the chance.

Elizabeth has always encouraged me to pursue writing. I have written little poems and stories all of her life, and prior, as a hobby or just for fun. She has been the inspiration for many of my writings and she has been one of my biggest fans. When I stumbled across the *Chicken Soup for the American Idol Soul* writing contest it seemed to be the perfect opportunity. With my newfound realization, Elizabeth and I had watched the *American Idol* series together, sometimes laughing until we cried and sometimes in utter amazement at the talent. All of those household chores and responsibilities were cast aside to share something that Elizabeth immensely enjoyed. And, obviously, I immensely enjoyed the time with Elizabeth.

Much to my surprise, I did win first prize in the contest. The prize included two tickets to see the two finale shows of *American Idol* at the Nokia Theatre in Los Angeles. Again, I thought of my realization and knew that Elizabeth would be extremely delighted to be in Los Angeles for the finale. So, we did something that we have never done and added to some of that spontaneity by allowing Elizabeth to miss a week of school. Off we headed to L.A.!

Toward the end of our very exciting trip, Elizabeth happily said, "Now I can cross another thing off my life list. I wanted to visit Los Angeles and we did!"

I guess you can say that my realization that I was wasting time on the wrong things, when I could have been sharing time with my daughter, has become a resolution after all. Now my resolution is to see Elizabeth cross items one by one off her life list and being able to share each and every special moment. Who cares about the dust bunnies?

~Lil Blosfield

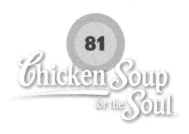

81

To See The World

Arriving at one goal is the starting point to another.
~John Dewey

It started in kindergarten. I made my resolution—I am going to see the world!

I was always curious about the globe and the many volumes of the *World Book Encyclopedia* in our house. I would climb up to reach them and take them off the shelves to peek. I learned a new big word... continents.

"We live in a Melting Pot." I remember hearing that and that I lived in... North America.

I noticed maps of oceans, countries, boundaries, lakes, and people. I began drawing pictures of the many different people who had come from all over to live in the United States.

I wanted to go to all seven continents!

Through travel, education, and amazing opportunities that came my way, I began to see the world.

In South America, I walked through rainforests with mountains, animal life, and vegetation, and... it really rained! Sopping wet, I heard talk that rainforests are disappearing.

Africa has a lot of languages among the people who live in cities and villages. We need to provide opportunities to lessen poverty and help to feed the families in the disadvantaged communities.

In Europe, I found out that Big Ben is not a giant person. Going to the top of the Eiffel Tower, and riding on a gondola in Venice were exciting and fun.

"Passengers, someone has lost something," announced the pilot on my flight to Australia. As we all looked around, he continued, "Laura has lost... her birthday." So on my way to "The Land Down Under," I experienced traveling through different time zones and going from summer to winter. The pilot tipped the plane a little so passengers could have a glance at The Great Barrier Reef.

Asia was special when I became intrigued with the pandas. And then, in Thailand, it was the elephants. I went to "elephant camp" and watched the elephants learn team-building as they stacked logs into place. I went on a raft, and through the trees I could hear locals singing as they rode their elephants in the villages. Then, to see elephants play in the water and spray like a carwash was a chance to realize... that animals big and small need the help of people like you and me.

"Think green." I began hearing scientists predict that global warming is underway. My resolution began to evolve; I needed to not just hear the words, but to learn more about "going green."

I was speaking on a ship in South America when offered the opportunity to fly to Antarctica. It took me only one second to say... Yes!

My resolution to visit all seven continents became — reality!

I didn't need my alarm clock to ring at 3 A.M. I was daydreaming about my resolution... to see the world. I didn't even know some of the passengers who loaned me clothes. I put on seven layers, two wool hats, two pairs of gloves, men's boots over my boots, and... felt like a stuffed sausage.

Antarctica is not an easy place to get to! I boarded a small (very small) plane with a veterinarian who was a scientist and wildlife expert. While in route, depending on the weather, the pilot wasn't sure if we could land. And... we did! The veterinarian explained she had prepared twenty times before her first landing in Antarctica.

I could barely walk and waddled... like a penguin. The land on Ardley Island looked to me like what space might look like. I could see red, orange and yellow growths amidst gray, brown, and green on the rocks.

I was with Chilean, Russian and German scientists who were all getting along. I kept thinking, why can't the world get along?

The wind blew as we explored. I put on a big life jacket and got into a little Zodiac. I never thought about the freezing waters below me and the real danger. The Zodiac glided along and the ice water splashed up. Brrrr.

I saw astounding scenery, wildlife, and penguins. As I was helped out of the Zodiac, I was told, "Penguins have the right of way." It was like a foreign land — the land of penguins. I waddled just like them and they were just all so busy. Penguin moms were near the water and some were ready to return to their families. It was like seeing the line to get into the after-Thanksgiving sale at a department store.

Dads who had been sitting on the eggs hatched two babies each. Each had his own distinct sounds, the pitch or yelp that they talked with. I talked to them too. I couldn't help it! "Don't worry; your Mommy will be here soon." The mouths of the young just reunited were open and being fed. The others were waiting... with hope. Some were lying on their bellies and sliding down a slope while their elders watched for predators. My heart went out to them when I remembered the penguin movies I have seen and the stories of woe.

I returned in the Zodiac to the small airstrip. They say Antarctica is the coldest and windiest continent. I decided that layer number seven could come off as I became somewhat comfortable. Wrong! I unbuttoned my jacket and rounded the corner on the path to the airplane. That was when the Antarctic wind blew and I was too cold and windblown to refasten my coat. The strong wind force was against me, I was moving in the wrong direction! A naturalist helped me make it to the plane. Ahhhhhhh, ascending the stairs to warmth. I had fulfilled a dream; my life's resolution had come true.

It took visiting all seven continents to fulfill my resolution to visit the globe.

Now a new resolution waits for me. To help!

I used to hear, "You can't protect what you don't know." The one thing I've learned in all my travels is that the planet needs our help right now. We all need to find a way to help in "going green."

My childhood resolution has been achieved and I have discovered a new, more important resolution.

How we can all help to save our earth?!

~Gail Small

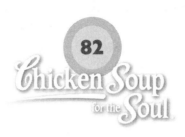

Chicken Soup
for the Soul

I Wasn't Expected to Succeed

Don't aim for success if you want it; just believe in yourself,
do what you love and believe in, and it will come naturally.
~David Frost

It was the seventies. I was a poor kid from a large family, and a girl to boot.

To make matters worse, I was a mediocre student. Math concepts eluded me, as did foreign language and science. I wasn't musically inclined, either, though I did have a bit of creativity going for me. Being creative, however, labeled me a cheat in ninth grade when I got the right answers but the wrong equations in algebra class. Because I couldn't breathe in gym class and lagged behind the rest of the group, I was labeled "slow and lazy." No one ever suggested the right label might have been "asthmatic." Being too shy to shower in front of the rest of the class, I was written up time and time again as disobedient.

They expected a truant student, so after a while, I complied. I was a rebel, a ne'er do well. I wasn't up to standards. I certainly wasn't expected to succeed.

My future plans included becoming a reporter and author, possibly an elementary teacher, but when I relayed that to my counselor, I discovered we didn't see eye to eye. The word "college" wasn't even mentioned during our "career directive" meeting, but words like "waitress" and "clerk" and "cleaning lady" were batted about the room like ping pong balls, all landing in my lap... and me without the proverbial paddle.

"I like to write," I said timidly. "I was thinking I'd like to be a reporter or an author... maybe write books for children."

His eyebrows rose and he nodded, considering....

And then... now that my portfolio had finally been opened... he had a brainstorm. I might consider becoming a secretary! After all, I had taken all of the secretarial classes, and I was a good writer. My spelling ability was above average. My shorthand was good; my office equipment skills were up to par.

"I don't really want... any... jobs like that," I replied.

He looked at me then, and smiled kindly. "I'd like to send you in a direction that would be more fitting with the skills you have," he said as he leaned back in his chair. "Of course... you'll want to get married and raise a family."

My heart fell. Regardless of what he was saying, what I heard was that once again I wasn't expected to succeed. Disappointment grew in the pit of my stomach. I thanked him and told him I would think about it. But as I walked back down the hall to my classroom, my cheeks burned with humiliation.

I didn't blame him. Based on the page in front of him, and what he had known of me as a student, he had tried to advise me to the best of his ability. What he didn't know was that the page in front of him wasn't me. None of my teachers knew the real me — they'd never taken the time to find out who I was. Or was it that I'd never believed in myself to begin with?

After graduation, I did exactly as my counselor suggested. As one of three secretaries in the Applied Mechanics and Engineering Science Department at the University of Michigan, I helped six professors help their students make their dreams become reality. Every day for two long years I watched other young adults make their way through college.

Within a few short years following high school, I had become a statistic.

At the age of twenty, I married my high school sweetheart and started my family. I didn't think about my career again until I had two toddlers underfoot and a burning need to discover what my mission on this planet was supposed to be. At the time, my husband was enrolled in evening classes to further his education, so college for me was out of the question.

Because of our family situation, I knew whatever I decided to do would have to be inexpensive and attainable from the comfort of my own home. By a stroke of sheer luck, I found what I was looking for in the back of a magazine. The Institute of Children's Literature was looking for people who wanted to write children's books. By cutting corners, I managed to save enough money to take the course by mail.

Since I was also the Girl Scout Leader for my daughters' troop, I double-dipped assignments and duties whenever possible. Class assignments revolved around troop activities and vice versa. After finishing each essay, I'd address one copy to the school and pop it in the mailbox, and slip a second copy beneath the door of the local newspaper. You can't imagine how pleased I was when the articles began showing up in the paper with my byline attached.

Of course, there was no pay, but I was ecstatic!

In March, 1986, the same month I finished my classes and delivered my third child, the publisher of the newspaper and I bumped into one another as I slipped yet another story beneath his door. He hired me on the spot and within two years I was named editor.

For seventeen years, I made a living as a journalist and photographer for *The Milan News* and several other local papers, including *The Ann Arbor News*. Since then, I have been published in more newspapers, magazines, and online newsletters and print anthologies than I can count. To date, my name also appears on the cover of eight books.

Finally—the hard way—my dreams have become my reality.

I realize now that the responsibility to succeed belonged to me, not my teachers or counselors. I was the one who hadn't expected me to succeed. I now also know it really doesn't matter what anyone else thinks about me or my abilities, it's what I think that matters. All anyone ever has to do in order to succeed is "expect" to succeed. These days I expect miracles every day of my life, and every day of my life I receive them.

~Helen Kay Polaski

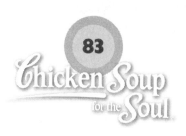

To Meet a Prince

But there's nothing half so sweet in life as love's young dream.
~Thomas Moore

If the need to tell our stories is what connects us, imagination is what renders those stories unique. Imagination fuels resolutions and shapes dreams. So it was for me at twelve years old when I first heard a newscast about Charles, Prince of Wales.

I was staying the week with my grandparents, as I did several times every summer. I quite simply adored my grandparents, and for months looked forward to our weeks together. I always loved suppertime best, not only because Gram let me plan the meal from her repertoire of delicious home cooking, but also because Granddad came home, smelling faintly of whatever mechanical things he did at the pump supply store where he worked. Every night while we ate, the three of us watched the evening news on the tiny black-and-white television in the corner of their kitchen, and that's where I learned of Charles. My imagination went into overdrive as I thought about how magical his life must be. I resolved then and there to someday meet a prince.

After supper, I could always be found on the swing in my grandparents' yard while Granddad went about his outside chores. The swing was my prime place for daydreaming, and on that night, my imagination didn't let me down. "Just how would this prince-meeting come about?" I asked myself. The story went something like this: first, I would fashion a new wardrobe—shimmery white ballgowns and satin slippers, dresses in every rainbow shade. Second, I would leave my Midwestern hometown. Princes didn't live in such unimportant places. I would cross the country, cross the Atlantic....

"Hey, there," Granddad said as he joined me on the swing, which had to slow down to accommodate his long legs. He took out his handkerchief and wiped the sweat from his brow. He had been weeding the garden, and the sultry night air hugged us like one of Gram's prized quilts. "What'cha thinking?" he asked me.

I didn't dare tell him about my exciting unfolding story. No, instead, we talked of... fireflies. A silly conversation, considering what princes must discuss, but I had to humor my granddad. Before long, as we sat watching the little bugs blink on and off in front of our eyes, our firefly talk prompted stories of his childhood, which invariably led to stories of his trips to Germany or stories of when he used to work at the railroad company.

That night, I lay in the heat of my grandparents' upstairs bedroom, listening to the drone of the window fan mixed with the song of balladeer crickets. The house smelled like summer and spent sunshine, and the scent from supper of Gram's vinegary lettuce.

Finally... I could get back to my story.

So where was I? Oh, yes, crossing the Atlantic. Maybe the prince would actually be the one to do that. He was a helicopter pilot, you know, and it might just be that he'd like to see the world from this side of the ocean. Okay, but that still didn't explain how I met him, I thought, yawning as my eyelids closed. Gosh, that lettuce had sure tasted good...

The next night, I couldn't wait to scurry out to the swing. My imagination was still spinning, my tale taking on a life of its own, though admittedly tripped up a bit over that little how-I-met-the-prince part. Well, I'd come back to that, I decided, choosing instead to work out the part where I'm introduced to all of England. Of course it would be on the evening news. Mr. Cronkite would surely be impressed. As an admired architect, I was in the process of rebuilding Windsor Castle, where the prince and I... no, no... scratch that. I've just come back from Africa, um, Antarctica... where, while on a polar bear expedition... sigh. As a world-famous doctor, I'm in England to perform surgery....

The sound of thunder startled me from my fantasy. I gazed up to darkening storm clouds, waved to Granddad as he made his ump-teenth pass across the lawn with his lawnmower. He was preoccupied that night, his goals centered on getting the grass cut before the rain moved in, the strawberries picked before the mosquitoes got hungry. When he finished the yard, I ran to help him in the strawberry patch, swatting mosquitoes as raindrops began to fall. "Your gram's gonna be mad that you're good and soaking wet," he said, a feisty twinkle in his eye.

I laughed, delighting in the rain, all thoughts of the prince forgotten.

Gram studied us with mock sternness when we entered the kitchen. "Look at you both," she scolded. "You're good and soaking wet."

Granddad just winked at me.

That week rolled on, fading into the next summer and the next, until one summer's night I'm sharing dinner with my husband as we watch the evening news. We've built a good life for ourselves; we've been married more than thirty years, having fallen in love when we worked together at a movie theater. My husband is a wonderful man, though he sometimes gets preoccupied with things like cutting the grass before the rain moves in or weeding the flower garden before the mosquitoes bite. He has a passion for baseball and leaves his socks in strange places. He also has a passion for our children, for our family and friends, for me.

Suddenly, my attention is drawn to the TV and a story about Prince Charles on a trip to Scotland with his sons. I smile, feeling a touch of embarrassment. Funny, that old resolution: It burns in my memory like those long-ago fireflies that brightened my nights and then flew away. Funny how ballgowns gave way to ballgames, satin slippers to jeans and tennis shoes. Oh, and that little how-I-met-the-prince part? I met him at a movie theater and we fell in love....

~Theresa Sanders

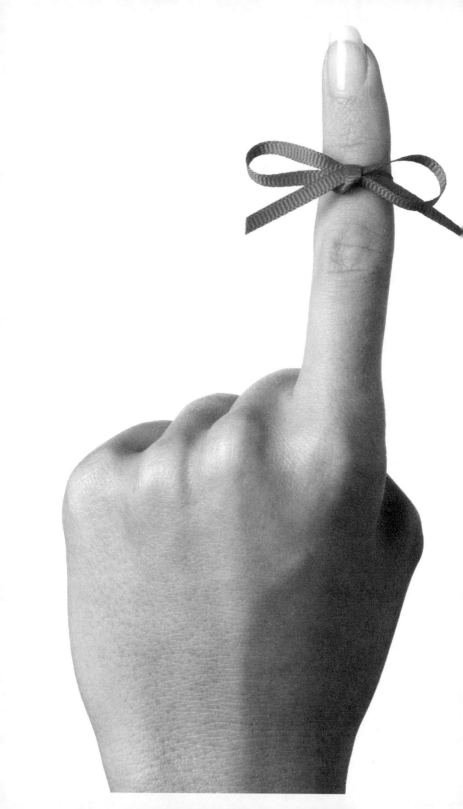

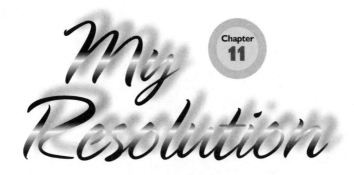

Chapter
11

I Actually Like This!

It's so hard when I have to, and so easy when I want to.

~Annie Gottlier

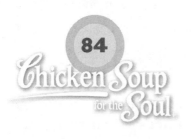

A Daily Practice in Gratitude

As each day comes to us refreshed and anew, so does my gratitude renew itself daily. The breaking of the sun over the horizon is my grateful heart dawning upon a blessed world.
~Adabella Radici

I am a list lover. Lists organize me and keep me that way. Each morning over coffee, I scribble the day's "To Do" items on a lined pad. What I don't accomplish one day, I add to the top of my list for the next. I love my lists. I'd be a chaotic mess without them. So it wasn't a stretch that my 2008 New Year's resolution was to keep a daily gratitude list.

I planned to write down three things a day that expressed my appreciation and love for the people and things around me. What began as a simple mission failed miserably by the end of January. Some days, I could not come up with one single thing for which to be grateful. On other days, I resented what my life withheld from me, instead of acknowledging the good already in it. What started as a positive exercise turned into a mental list of countless complaints and worries. Temporary family concerns and financial woes had turned me into an ungrateful sourpuss.

A stranger changed all that for me. I noticed her one early spring morning as I walked toward the grocery store's entrance. She wrestled unsuccessfully to free a shopping cart from a line of them snaked along the wall. She did this with one hand, while the other carefully held the wrist of her bald daughter, who looked to be around four years old.

I shook my head in disgust as I watched two able-bodied men barge past her, each with a cell phone in his ear. I grappled with the stubborn cart, liberating it from the others, and then stepped aside, waiting for her to load the small girl into its seat. As she hoisted up her frail, sick daughter, I couldn't help but notice the child weighed next to nothing. Her pasty skin and swollen face made her sunken eyes appear bigger than they were, revealing a wealth of pain I could only image. She reached out to her mother and, for the briefest instant, I witnessed an exchange of love so pure pass between them that my throat tightened and I had to look away. That grateful woman turned to me and with a smile stretched wide across her drawn and tired face said, "Thanks. You're a life saver!"

Suddenly my troubles seemed petty and small. I experienced a major attitude change. I've had that happen before but it never lasted. This time I was determined to hold on to that shift and absorb it. The next morning my gratitude list took on a life of its own. I allowed not one negative thought as I quickly filled a page of my "To Do" pad with the abundance in my life and moved to another. I listed good health, a comfortable home, a car that works, and family and friends to love. Eventually, I had to find another pad to fill.

Days later, I picked up a beautiful journal with a ribbon book-mark, and I kept it on my nightstand. It became my gratitude journal. If I'm too tired to list at least three things I am grateful for before I crawl into bed at night, I make it a point, after I open my eyes each morning, to jot down three positives about my life. I do this even before my feet hit the floor. It only takes a moment and what a wonderful way to start the day. If I can't remember three things from the night before, I begin with what I feel now. I'm grateful for cool cotton bedsheets, sunshine streaming through my window, the way my body feels when I stretch my toes to the end of the mattress. It's easy to find things to be grateful for when you pay attention to the world around you.

The shopping cart lady reminded me that the things you believe you are not receiving from life, you are not giving out yourself. Whenever I think people are not offering me what I would like from them—respect, kindness, help, recognition, attention—I give it to them first. The results from a simple act of kindness are astounding. When I tell my husband that I'm grateful for his support, I get support from him. When I praise my children for their successes, sometimes I get praise in return.

My initial resolution to keep a daily gratitude list that would change my life backfired in the best possible way. Instead of it making me happy, I use it as a wonderful tool to remind me to notice the beauty all around me. In order for this to happen, I became a daily giver. I'm the one who smiles first as I hold the door open for a woman pushing a baby carriage, offer a sincere compliment to the person behind the checkout counter, and wish a good morning to fellow walkers on the park trail.

Once I recognized you could not receive what you do not give, most of my days became joyful instead of stress-filled. The realization that true abundance comes from within, not outside you, started with a smile. A stranger's smile.

Tomorrow I need to shop for a new gratitude journal. Mine is full.

~Sarah Jo Smith

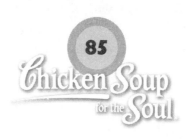

Eating Healthy If It Kills Us

> *As a child my family's menu consisted of two choices: take it or leave it.*
> ~Buddy Hackett

Following a bout with breast cancer back in 1999, I made a resolution to change my deplorable eating habits to a healthy, plant-based program of nutrition. This meant, of course, that I would have to convert my husband and two teenaged children as well.

Their reaction to my first meal?

"What's this stuff on my plate?" My son, Aaron, circled the dinner table, eyes narrowed suspiciously, lip threatening to curl.

"Which stuff might that be?" I asked, with an innocent lift of my eyebrow.

"This weed-looking thing here next to this... this... what IS this thing the weed is sitting next to?"

Ignoring him for the moment, I called my husband, Fred, and my daughter, Summer, to the table.

Summer galloped into the room. "Geez, Mom, it's about time, I am STARVING!" Stopping suddenly in her tracks, anticipatory smile fading, nostrils twitching, "What's that smell?"

"Dinner," I said.

Moving to where Aaron hovered anxiously above his place setting, she stood beside him, peering down at her plate. "Why is there a weed on my plate?" she demanded. "And what's this thing it's sitting next to?"

"It's not a weed, it's kale, for crying out loud," I explained. "It's a cruciferous vegetable."

"Cruciferous is another way of saying it's some weird thing she found in the backyard!" Aaron interpreted for his sister.

"That's disgusting."

"I did not get it from the backyard. I got it at the health food store," I said, turning for support to Freddie, who had just come on the scene.

"What's that smell?" he asked.

He joined Summer and Aaron at the table. "Why is...?" Anticipating the rest of the question, Summer said, "It's not a weed; it's Kale. Mom found it in the backyard."

"Just sit down and eat," I sighed.

My family deposited themselves in their appropriate places and reluctantly picked up forks. Fred prodding the main course and asked, "What's this?"

"Yeah, that's what I want to know," Aaron said. "It doesn't look like food."

Summer nodded a vigorous agreement.

"It's a veggie burger," I said, squirting catsup over the patty.

Freddie examined his up close, "Looks like brown gravel, bird-seed and oatmeal," he pronounced.

Summer, nudging her mashed potatoes protectively away from her patty, asked, "Have we been bad?"

I shook my head in exasperation, "It tastes just like hamburger, only it's good for you." Cutting a small piece with my fork, I popped it into my mouth. My family watched skeptically. I chewed, and then swallowed, a bright, contented smile on my lips.

They weren't buying it.

"Eat your weeds," I muttered, pointing a threatening fork. "It's not negotiable. This family is going to eat healthy if it kills us."

Groaning collectively, with expressions resembling those of prisoners facing a firing squad, they began to eat.

"See," I said, "It's not that bad."

Aaron and Summer grimaced, each alternating small bites of pseudo-burger with large gulps of iced tea. Freddie merely shrugged, concentrating most of his attention on his mashed potatoes. A few minutes later, Aaron's expression brightened.

"Hey, what's for dessert?"

I couldn't help myself. "Tofu pudding!"

"Ewwwwwwwww!"

"Just kidding."

Sometimes my family has no sense of humor.

So, that initial dinner was my first clue that maybe the whole "healthy eating," "healthy living" resolution was going to take some serious getting used to.

Even I, as enthusiastic as I was about getting back to nature, was dismayed to discover what any honest health food zealot will admit, albeit under torture: If it's good for you, it will probably resemble something found floating on the top of your backyard fishpond, and will taste of barkdust.

But, on the upside, that was nearly nine years ago, and no one in the family has died from offended taste buds. Fred has decided that chickens grown free range taste pretty much the same as the ones grown in a pen. Summer has admitted that she actually likes kale. Aaron—well, what can I say? He's living on his own now and I'm pretty sure the closest thing to a vegetable going into his mouth is a French fry.

And me? I discovered a green tea that doesn't taste like pond scum, as well as some healthy recipes that are actually good. All in all, I'd have to say that even though I've failed at many of the resolutions I've made over the years... this is one I've managed to keep.

~Tina Wagner Mattern

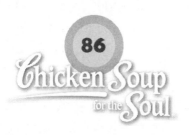

A Commitment to Play Dolls

It is much easier to become a father than to be one.
~Kent Nerburn

Of course I cried out. Transitions are always painful: Birth, death, trading in my beloved sports car for the family sedan.

And this was every bit as anguishing, as irrevocable. It was the day my daughter stared up at me with her big, pleading eyes and said, "Daddy, will you play dolls with me?"

Like most fathers, I was lost. Nature hadn't prepared me for anything like this. I stood there motionless, wishing I were somewhere, anywhere else.

Legos? Sure. Nintendo? No problem. But dolls? Suddenly I was clueless.

My lack of knowledge on the subject of dolls is really nobody's fault. It was simply a lousy little wrong that's been handed down from one man to the next in my family, like my great-grandfather's rusty old pocket watch that nobody ever hated quite enough to toss.

Throughout the ages, men have never been properly schooled in the fine art of playing dolls. I waited until I was forty years old to play with my first doll. When I was a kid, I though they were dumb. Besides, my sister was bigger than me and wouldn't let me play with her dolls.

I still think playing with dolls is dumb. But my four-year-old daughter, Emily, loves them. She plays with her Barbie dolls every day. Since I want to be a good father, and because Emily and I don't get to spend much time together, I resolved to learn.

The first thing I noticed when I sat down to play was the absence of boy dolls. There was Dance Moves Barbie, Tropical Splash Barbie, Bubble Angel Barbie, Baywatch Barbie, and Hot Skatin' Barbie, but not one Ken doll in the whole collection. Only Barbie.

There's a good reason for that, I suppose. Little girls spend a lot of time dressing and undressing their dolls, pulling off fuchsia miniskirts and halter tops, putting on stewardess uniforms and gold-sequined gowns. Wardrobes for every occasion.

What self-respecting boy doll would want to go through that?

Emily chose Butterfly Princess Barbie to play with. I got Slumber Party Barbie.

"There you go," she said, thrusting the doll into my hand. There you go. As simple as that. For long minutes I sat there, staring at the doll.

"Um... ah.... What would you like to play?" I asked.

Emily sighed, "I already told you, daddy," she said. "We're playing dolls."

Eventually, I began to get the hang of it. We dressed our Barbie dolls in designer clothes, drove them to the mall in a hot red convertible, changed their clothes, and drove them home... where we changed their clothes again. And again. We changed Barbie's clothes more times than I can remember. We changed Barbie's clothes until my fingers went numb.

There was something special about sitting cross-legged on the floor with my daughter, snacking on Goldfish crackers and juice boxes, and watching her change Barbie from her spring ensemble to her summer ensemble.

I took on this doll play thing with a passion born of a higher consciousness. I labored at understanding colors. I worked on coordinating my fashion. I accepted the challenge. I entered Barbie Country, tamed the maelstrom, and emerged laughing....

Well, I did okay.

Most of the clothes I put on Slumber Party Barbie didn't go together. When I dressed my doll in a purple blouse and orange shorts, Emily looked at me and pulled a face.

"Da-dee!" she said, "Those things don't match!" Dressing a doll properly is, to my daughter, the cornerstone of civilization. Consider all the things that can be improved just by wearing clothes that match!

Another thing I enjoyed about playing dolls is that you can make your doll do whatever you want it to. My daughter made her Barbie doll work as a fashion model and then go shopping for clothes. I made my doll stay home and clean house. What can I say? I'm an old-fashioned kind of guy.

I was about to put my doll to work mopping the kitchen floor when a voice of sanity cautioned me that this was the wrong tack. Actually, it was Emily giving me a funny look. The kind of look her mother gives me when I watch too much football on the weekends. So I let my doll go out and get a job... as a short order cook. Another reason I like playing dolls is because in doll land any and all problems can be cleared up quickly. Marital problems? C'mon, let's make up! Overdue bills? Heck, just pay 'em off! What? You wrecked the car? Don't worry, honey, the mechanic will fix it!

It's enough to make a father want to take up residence in doll land.

Eventually, though, Emily grew tired of watching me send Barbie off to her job at McDonald's and suggested that we do something else.

"Like what?" I asked, secretly hoping she would consider sacking the whole Barbie doll game for the Rams/49ers game, which was about to start.

"We can comb Barbie's hair!" said my daughter. "It will be fun."

To be truthful, combing Barbie's hair was not much fun. Actually, it was an event on the thrill scale equal only to watching Walter Cronkite get his nose hairs clipped. Besides, I wasn't very good at it. I accidentally kept pulling Barbie's bleached blond hair out in big clumps. I was leaving an ever-growing trail of incompetence behind me.

After we finished combing hair, we put our Barbie dolls back in the convertible and took them for a ride. My daughter's idea of a ride was more like a demolition derby.

"Careful," I told her. "Don't wreck that car. It might have to go back in the shop for another thirty seconds."

Emily and I played dolls for several hours (or at least it felt that long) and I must admit, for a complete novice I wasn't all that bad. I'll do you a favor and not tell you how I dressed Barbie for the prom. Or the beach.

"Da-dee! She can't go to the beach without a top!" she laughed, sunshine beaming from her sweet face once more. I bent down and kissed her soft cheek.

What did I learn from all of this? I learned that there is a fine father/daughter relationship that can be developed while doing things like playing Barbie dolls.

And I'm looking forward to our next session with a sense of... what? Foreboding? Anxiety? The willies? Oh, yes, now I remember: anticipation.

~Timothy Martin

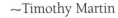

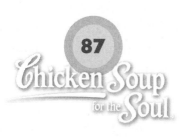

87

Hybrid Harmony

Kilometers are shorter than miles.
Save gas, take your next trip in kilometers.
~George Carlin

I feel like I'm reborn. I'm still a forty-year-old homemaker in Greenwich, CT, with three kids, a husband, and a dog. But a psychic weight has been lifted from my shoulders and I've transcended the suburban jungle around me. I have a spring in my step and my neck muscles are finally relaxed. Did I find a miracle diet to melt all traces of fat? A yoga guru to transport me to spiritual ecstasy? Definitely not. I'm exactly the same person as before, only now I'm enlightened.

I'm driving a new car, in fact a whole new class of car (at least among my Mommy friends). Since I had my first child ten years ago I've been driving big cars, the kind that could go head-to-head with a truck should they ever collide. I've driven SUVs made by Lexus, Mercedes, Volvo, and BMW. I was a suburban stereotype—driving my luxury SUV with a Blackberry headset in my ear and a Starbucks at my side. But those days of excess are over. I've found a new guilt-free indulgence and it's the Toyota Prius. The egg-shaped compact hybrid car is now our preferred mode of transportation.

In the pick-up line at school, other moms ask doubtfully, "Does that really fit everybody?"

"Yes" I answer "and hockey bags too."

They pause to ponder whether I'm an environmental zealot or

just trying to be trendy. What they're also calculating is whether they could survive in a car where children actually sit next to one another. The idea of those little humans in close proximity—with the ability to pinch, push and spit on their neighbor—does not conjure a peaceful ideal. Instead, they envision tangled limbs, piercing screams and an occasional Gameboy hurled through the air. Better to separate the children into their own territories, with individual entertainment centers and feeding stations. That way moms can drive and talk undisturbed on their Bluetooth headsets. Why give up the fortress of an SUV for a silly blob of a car that could probably be crushed by an Escalade?

For years, I'd eyed the Prius. Its body puzzled me—was it adorable or ugly? And as a former corporate attorney, I questioned its performance prowess. How could this hybrid achieve 45 mpg when all others could barely break 30? Surely the car must have a fatal flaw that would be revealed in a class action suit someday. I imagined a plaintiff telling the jury that after hitting a pothole, his Prius catapulted into the air and was crushed like an accordion. It's not a car, you see, just an aluminum-covered balloon. But my cynical fantasies never materialized. Everywhere I went I saw more of these creatures prowling the road. The rest of the world was buying into this trend and apparently enjoying the experience.

One day, I secretly went for a test drive. It was surprisingly smooth, more of a sedan than the tin can I expected. When I reached the first traffic light, I felt like a toddler strapped in a stroller looking up at my surroundings. But my perspective soon adjusted. I began to pity all those supersized SUVs. They looked like overworked horses—Clydesdales who'd been carting their loads far too long. Their engines gunned even when standing still. The exhaust pouring out would nauseate anyone nearby. But their drivers—ensconced in their soundproof cockpits yards away—were oblivious. They never saw or smelled any of this waste, as they drove from errand to activity and back again. Everyone says they're in favor of clean air, but have they looked to see what's coming out of their own tailpipe?

Coming from the world of hermetically-sealed, tank-like

vehicles, converting to a Prius has been a life-altering experience for me. (I realize that I'm on the tail end of the hybrid trend, but we're not known for being cutting-edge in Greenwich). The first thing I noticed when the ignition turned on was Silence, even with the windows open. No spewing sounds of fuel combustion. A quiet hush. Does anyone remember what that sounds like? In a life filled with chaos and noise, silence is a true luxury, a calming force. I began to think this car might be the antidote to my harried existence. The next big difference is that driving a Prius feels more like gliding.

The thrill of being in this stream-lined Jetsonesque car started to take hold. When I finally drove my own model off the lot, I felt exhilarated—and liberated. My conscience was free from the shackles of the monster truck and its toxic carbon emissions. I was doing my part to save the environment and parking would be a whole lot easier too.

The ultimate surprise was how quickly my children fell for the car too. At first they said it was "weird" but curiosity overcame them. After the second day of shuttling about, they were excited to be in the Prius. It's not just the novelty of the car that appeals to them, but something deeper and more personal. The Prius has none of the "child-friendly" gadgets that are now standard in family cars—no individual DVD screens or headsets. But my kids never noticed this absence. Instead their joy seems to come from within—the voice that says I want to see the world at eye level and be recognized as an equal. This car matches their own body size, and makes them feel substantial. Whether they realize it or not, the smaller size also brings us closer together—literally and spiritually. Snuggling in a space where the only entertainment choices are conversation or music is a newly-discovered pleasure. It recharges our connections with each other and makes us whole again.

My generation of women grew up before SUVs and minivans were invented, but now we accept these as a necessary part of family life. It's a classic example of groupthink. If everyone else has one, then I need one too. We can just as easily unravel this knot by thinking ourselves in another direction. People seem to postpone choosing a hybrid car because the perfect model isn't yet available. They expect something that looks and feels just like their current car, only with the fuel-efficiency of a motorbike. That mentality is exactly what allows car manufacturers to avoid changing their product lines. They count on the fact that consumers dislike change.

I propose that consumers buying family cars make their voices heard by choosing smaller, hybrid cars. The overscaled, gas-guzzling vehicles of the past decade are relics of an era of self-absorption. We are now fully informed about the consequences of burning copious amounts of gas. Not only will air quality plummet and global warming rise, but foreign policy will be dictated by gasoline addiction. We cannot pretend to be helpless in this struggle. A hybrid car may not solve the entire problem, but it is certainly a step in the right direction. And the added benefits of family harmony and spiritual liberation are priceless. From my own experience, I conclude that everyone should rethink their wheels, and when it comes to driving the family, a smaller and cleaner car just feels better.

~Alexandra Bergstein

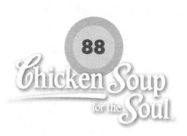

88

I'm Not a Dirty Hippie

You have to leave the city of your comfort and go into the wilderness
of your intuition. What you'll discover will be wonderful.
~Alan Alda

I remember the first time I mentioned to my husband that I wanted to "go green"—or, at least "greener." His response was a stream of water, shooting from his nose and choked laughter. "Ash," he said, "you are so funny."

"I mean it." I pressed on, "I want to start cloth-diapering Lorelei." His eyes grew to the size of silver dollar coins. "Cloth diapers?" he asked. "Isn't that like... back in the day? Oh man. There is NO way I'm changing cloth diapers. NO way."

I nodded and went back to my corner, victoriously, to resume my research. To me, I had won. He hadn't exactly said "No," after all. He had just said that he wouldn't be changing cloth diapers. I simply knew that I wanted the best for our new baby, Lorelei. I knew that it was up to us to protect her—and for me, there was no turning back.

And, so it began—my resolution to live a greener life. My husband was behind me, and that meant the world to me—regardless of whether I had to drag him there. At least he was there. The diapers came in and my husband was delighted to see that they were nothing like the diapers of yesteryear that he'd imagined with horror. There would be no swishing in toilets and gagging—not even I was up for that mess. No, these diapers came with a waterproof outer shell and snaps instead of pins. We were well on our way.

What had begun as a journey for cloth diapers suddenly became a full-scale endeavor. The research for cloth diapers had uncovered some disturbing news about children's skincare products, which in turn led us to look at our own skincare products. My husband had had enough. "You won't turn me into a dirty hippie!" he said, when I merely suggested that his favorite brand of shampoo held more toxins than he wanted to know. I hadn't really meant that he should not wash his hair. I just wanted to find an alternative shampoo.

It took a while before my husband would even enter a health food store; his visits consisted mostly of him standing by the door or waiting in the car. It wasn't until our visit to a Whole Foods store that he began to see this new endeavor in a more positive light.

In awe, he looked upon the rows and rows of shelves. "It's... it's like a real grocery store!" he exclaimed, running to the candy aisle. Like a little boy lost in magic, the glow of something healthy, yet wonderfully tasty lured him in. He would pass by every other box, animatedly calling out to me, "Did you see this? What about this? This is so cool!" In a single trip, we had shattered one of the most amazing lies, "If it's good for you, it must taste bad."

Slowly, we began trying new products—with a lot of trial and error. We wanted products that we could not only afford, but that also worked and smelled good as well—to avoid smelling like "a dirty hippie" as my husband pointed out. After a lot of testing and trying, we began to find products that we could not only use, but that were more affordable than the products we previously used. We were amazed that we could find products that were better for us, for less. Well, I was, anyway. My husband was mostly glad that his new shampoo didn't smell like twigs.

One day, as I was browsing the shelves of our local health food store, a book about alternative healing caught my eye. I looked behind me, making sure my husband and daughter were occupied. I braced myself, preparing for any outlandish health schemes I might encounter. There weren't any. Inside the book were detailed alternative therapies for some of the symptoms we'd been suffering. Chronically. I couldn't believe it. For us, this could be the end of nights of lying awake in immense pain. And, it was.

What originally began as a mission to protect our daughter became a journey to improve our own lives. And it did, more than we could have ever imagined.

~Ashley Sanders

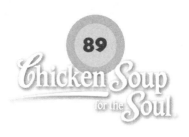

Spend, Spend, Spend

*The ability to simplify means to eliminate the unnecessary
so that the necessary may speak.*
~Hans Hofmann

It is the distinct responsibility of each of us to nurture and care for ourselves, our families, friends, communities and yes, that includes our planet! In order to do this, it is often necessary to spend, spend, spend!

During this troubled time in our economy, many of us have made resolutions to save. We will save money at the grocery stores by consciously looking for advertised promotions or using store coupons. We will save money on gas by making lists of our daily errands and plotting a course that will save us miles in unnecessary travel. Unplugging appliances that are not in use saves on electricity. And do we really need every TV turned on in the house?

I have found that in making a resolution to save, I have made the process more fun by deciding to "spend."

As I have pledged to save on lavish meals dining out, I have vowed to "spend" more time entertaining at home. By planning carefully thought-out menus and inviting special friends to share with us, we are able to "spend" quality time with loved ones.

I have vowed to save on gasoline by planning my destinations carefully and efficiently. However, instead of taking the same route each time, I alter it slightly. One street over one way or the other introduces me to new surroundings—sometimes a new discovery. Miles saved are well "spent."

I have made the decision to stay home at least one day each week. It has allowed me the sorely needed time to "spend" cleaning out closets, playing in my garden, and devoting some very precious time to my grandchildren.

Resolutions to save for the sake of our bank accounts, our economy, and our planet need not be tedious. Most everything we do in life can encompass an element of fun. While saving time, money, and energy we can enjoy the pleasure of "spending." In the eyes of your friends and family, your resolution to "spend" will be the best one you have ever made.

~Kristine Byron

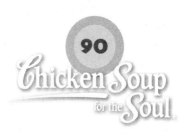

90

Learning to Appreciate My Father-In-Law

If you don't have time to do it right you must have time to do it over.
~Author Unknown

When it comes to long, grueling events, forget seven-day races and runs across the continent. For a real test of endurance, try remodeling a bedroom closet with your father-in-law.

That was the task my wife laid out for me when her parents came to visit. To be honest, I wasn't up to the job. It involved tearing out walls, rewiring outlets, moving pipes, spackling, painting, and moving a water heater. It also involved using precious time that I could better use watching my favorite team, the San Francisco Giants, play the Oakland As.

It's not that I don't like my father-in-law. He's a great guy. He's also a darn good carpenter. Put a saw and a piece of wood in Bob's hands, and cuts are ruler straight. When he joins two pieces of wood, they always fit perfectly. Bob believes in doing a job right. That's the part that troubled me. I have little patience for home improvement. When I hang a door, it hangs crooked. My cabinets resemble Picasso paintings, and my faucets spout water higher than Old Faithful. I don't care about craftsmanship. I just want to get the job done.

Realizing that my shoddy work habits wouldn't sit well with her dad, my wife asked me to mend my ways. At least temporarily. For the next week I was to forget about baseball and do exactly what my father-in-law asked me to. In short, I was to be the perfect helper.

There's nothing like a little home renovation to take your mind off the ball game.

My tactic on the first day was to watch a Giants game before Bob showed up. But my father-in-law arrived early, rushed to the bedroom, and immediately began taking measurements for the closet. He wanted to get right to work. I wanted to see how the team was doing, but I knew better.

I watched Bob closely. I fetched him wood, nails, and whatever else he needed. As he worked, I couldn't help but notice how long it took him to accomplish each task. Fifteen minutes to measure a board. Ten minutes to cut it. A full thirty minutes to decide where to install the plumbing. My emotions swelled and crashed like teenage mood swings. I wanted the job to go faster, but Bob's attention to detail was absolute.

It was as good a day as any to wean myself from my favorite pastime.

On the afternoon of the second day, my father-in-law asked me to cut a piece of wood. Black fear seized my organs. I wasn't a carpenter, but I did as instructed. Throwing caution to the wind, I snatched up the saw and started cutting. When Bob held the board in place, he shook his head. It was off by an inch.

"You have to do it again," he said.

"Why?" I asked.

"Because it doesn't fit right."

"So?" I said. Bob stared at me.

"You don't want the closet to turn out lopsided, do you?" It doesn't matter, I thought, biting my tongue. I just want the job to be done.

Four boards later, a miracle of sorts. My cut was straight. The board fit perfectly. But the job had taken its toll. My brain felt worn down to the knuckles. Worse yet, I had gone two full days without watching a single ball game.

The job moved slower than geological plate-shifting. One night I dropped into bed completely spent. I dreamed that Bob and I were working on the closet, and the World Series was about to begin. It was the Giants verses the Dodgers. I really wanted to watch the game, but Bob kept measuring a board for cutting. And then measuring it again. And again. And again. It was Board-Measuring Groundhog Day.

I kept saying, "It's good, Bob. It's fine." But he wouldn't listen. He just kept measuring and re-measuring the board.

I woke up screaming and in a cold sweat.

The next day, I complained to my wife. "You dad is taking way too long," I told her. "We should have finished the closet long ago."

"He's trying to do a good job," she replied. "If you were half the carpenter he is, maybe you'd understand."

Owwww! Kick a guy when he's down.

Time went into one of its long, slow, taffy-like stretches. The days blurred and I had to concentrate to keep them in sequence. Then an odd thing happened. At some point between the spackling and trim, I measured a board once, twice, three times. Without realizing what I was doing, I made sure the board was the proper length.

A strange combination of understanding and shame dawned on me, coming on like a rheostat-controlled light in a darkened theater. The closet was almost done and I was proud. It looked great.

Bob and I were just putting on the finishing touches when I noticed the doors still needed knobs.

"I'll put on those knobs," I told Bob.

"Why don't you watch the ball game," he said. "I'll finish up."

The words clotted on my tongue like lint from the dryer, but I actually replied, "That's okay, Bob. The game can wait."

~Timothy Martin

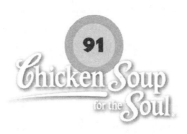

91

Prius in Seattle

*We shall require a substantially new manner of thinking
if mankind is to survive.*
~Albert Einstein

My husband pushes the "start" button on the dashboard of my new car. The only sound is the rubber tires on cement as we roll out onto the street. "Don't know why we waited so long to get a hybrid," he says with a grin bigger than a kid on his first bumper car ride. "All you do is boot it up—the computer takes care of the I.C.E."

"The what?" His new car lingo stumps me every time.

"You know, the internal combustion engine."

I roll my eyes. "Oh, that."

Several months ago, the guilt started seeping in. A string of alarming TV shows on global warming and the energy crisis had me thinking green. Lowering our carbon footprint seemed like a good way to get started, so I casually dropped the comment, "Maybe we should think about trading in my car for a hybrid."

Little did I know he would take the ball and run with it so quickly. This is the man who still reminisces over his life-long love affair with cars. Photos of his 1950s high school hot rods line the walls of his workshop. Next to them, a picture from his college days, standing proudly in tie-dyed T-shirt beside his '57 Volkswagen Beetle. To this day he bemoans the never-ending repair bills from our series of kid-safe late '70s Volvo station wagons. More recently he's entered a middle-aged phase with a penchant for big trucks and sport utilities.

But the past is past. He now claims our hybrid purchase is the best automobile decision of our lives and I have to agree. Owning a hybrid has been an interesting ride. Re-learning to drive and maximize the gas mileage in "my" new car has become "his" favorite pastime.

Who knew there was a world of Internet bloggers out there calling themselves "hyper-milers?" From Saskatoon to Arkansas, armed with his handle "Prius in Seattle," my husband culls information daily. Groundbreaking tips such as how overfilling your oil will lower your gas mileage. Idling at a stoplight and wasting even a drop of fuel is considered Prius-storic. And of course, there's that entire guy-type auto accessory shopping. Without leaving the comfort of your computer chair, you can purchase every thing from mud flaps to dashboard screen covers—deals the dealers don't even know about.

For the first mile or two out of the driveway my husband explains the importance of "good glide," also known as "feathering the throttle from full release." The critical thing here is keeping your speed under forty-two miles an hour. But that's just the beginning. His new Internet buddies have shared other gas-saving techniques like the "pulse and glide" and the "warp stealth." I'm thrilled.

"Watch the numbers," he says as we head towards the interstate. He points with glee to the MFD (Multi-Function Display) a device that looks like an electronic on-screen hamster cage complete with moving wheels, in the center of the dashboard.

Sure, I admit I was totally fascinated for the first few drives—those little spinning wheels simulating forward motion, the colored arrows flashing back and forth as the battery discharges and recharges. "Must be a lot of distracted Prius drivers on the road," I speculate, but he's quick with a comeback.

"We're more engaged in the whole driving process—that makes us even safer."

I'm mulling this over in my brain as we coast downhill.

The numbers at the bottom of the screen keep going up—from 46.5 to 49.4 miles per gallon. Hubby lets out a whoop as we get back on level terrain then flashes that silly grin again. "Can you believe it? I would have been thrilled to get half this mileage in our last car."

"Yeah sure, but look now." I can't help myself. As we make the next turn and start uphill the numbers are creeping back down, 47.3... 46.9.

Once again, he's fast with an answer. "I'm still working out a better route to the mall. Besides it's all about averaging, you know."

So it goes, our short hops around town are more often than not focused on fuel efficiency. Enjoying the view out the window on the way to the market or the movies has become secondary. But let's keep our priorities straight, I remind myself. Purchasing a PZEV (Partial-Zero Emission Vehicle) is a small start, but it's a commitment to going greener.

"Want to drive home?" my husband asks as we finish shopping and stroll back to the parking lot.

"I wouldn't dream of taking away your fun," I say. Besides, I know I'll never learn to meet his standards on feathering and gliding. Until we can afford another hybrid, it looks like the old gas-guzzling SUV in our garage is all mine. That is, if I can handle the guilt.

~Maureen Rogers

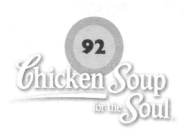

92

Blue, Brown & Green for Our Red, White & Blue

We do not inherit the earth from our ancestors;
we borrow it from our children.
~Native American Proverb

"You've got to be kidding," I raged. "I'm not going to separate our trash into three different containers. Forget it."

"It says here we'll be fined if we don't," my husband countered.

"Well, I'm not going to," I stubbornly replied. Chicken bones, potato peelings, cardboard cartons, plastic milk jugs; I put all of it together in one bag into one trashcan every night. That's the way I'd always done it, and that's the way I wanted to keep doing it. None of this fancy-schmancy sorting for me.

The flyer that came in the mail from our disposal company was colorful and enticing... a new recycling effort in our city; better for our landfills; less waste. Yeah, but what about my time? They wanted yard clippings in the green cart, recyclables in the blue one, and other trash in the brown one. All of this would take so much extra work. I tossed the brochure on top of the empty soup cans in the garbage.

The bins arrived on a Thursday a few weeks later. You could hear the new energy-efficient behemoth trucks lumbering down the street. With a whoosh and a screech, the truck stopped in front of each house and, using a mechanized lift, deposited a blue bin at the curb. Then the lift rode up the track to the top of the truck, grabbed a green bin, brought that one down, and repeated the process for a brown one. Three huge, 95 gallon plastic bins on rolling wheels now sat in front of every home on the block.

"I'm not happy about this," I complained to a neighbor as we started wheeling them one-by-one into our backyards. They had a large handle on the back and a smaller one in front for maneuverability, but to me they were anything but maneuverable. They were monsters.

"Me, neither," she said. "They're too big."

"Yeah, and wait until they're full. They'll not only be big, but heavy."

I wheeled the first one through our side gate and surveyed the spot where we used to keep two regular-sized trashcans. These monstrosities wouldn't fit in the old location. I moved a wire shelving unit where we kept gardening supplies, lugged the dog house from the dog's favorite corner and squeezed it in tight by the shed that held shovels and rakes. After more juggling, I managed to cram Big Blue, Big Green, and Big Brown next to the hoses and extra potting materials.

I stepped back and looked at them. "I hate these things," I mumbled to myself. They changed the way our backyard looked, like a ketchup stain on a white shirt.

That weekend we did some yard work. Weeds, dead pruned roses, some tree limbs cut down. "Where does this stuff go?" my husband asked. "Is this supposed to go in the green one?"

"I guess so. It says 'yard waste' on it," I replied.

"What about the dog droppings? Is that yard waste, too, or something else?"

"I don't know," I said with half a smile. "Should we put it in the brown one since it's the same color?"

"You got me."

We finally decided to keep the green one strictly for prunings and grass clippings. "Okay," I said, "that was an easy decision. Now what about this big blue giant? What goes in there?"

"The small print on the top says: cardboard, plastic, paper, glass bottles and cans."

"Well, we can put cardboard boxes in there from packages delivered to the house."

"Right," my husband said. "And how about newspapers after you read them?"

"Those I put out by the mailbox on trash day for the guys that drive around. I'd hate to stop helping them. I think they make a few bucks by turning them in or something."

"Okay, laundry detergent or plastic milk jugs, with the caps or lids off. And they say to wash out and flatten aluminum cans."

"No way. I have a hard enough time getting dinner ready without washing out a metal can before I throw it away."

"I'm just reading what it says. Don't jump all over me."

"I'm not, but this is ridiculous."

On trash collection day, I wheeled out Big Brown and Big Blue. There wasn't much in Big Green so I left that one behind until it had more in it. Big Brown was heavy and muscling it down the driveway and out to the curb made my muscles strain.

Time passed, and months later my husband stood in the kitchen after dinner. "What are you doing?" he said.

"Smashing this cardboard carton for Big Blue." I had it on the floor, with one foot holding it down while the other foot flattened the end.

"You, sorting trash?"

"Yes, and don't be so shocked. It doesn't take as much time as I thought."

"What happened to fussing about three separate containers?"

"I don't know. I guess I hated change. But now that I'm used to it, I love doing my part."

"That's my girl," my husband said, when he took me in his arms and hugged me. "And look at those muscles you're getting. Almost as big as mine."

"Not quite," I replied. "But here, use yours to take this stuff outside." I handed him the squashed cardboard and the rest of the garbage. "And make sure you put it in the right bin: Brown or Blue."

"Got it," he said with a wink. "A little blue, brown and green for our red, white and blue."

~B.J. Taylor

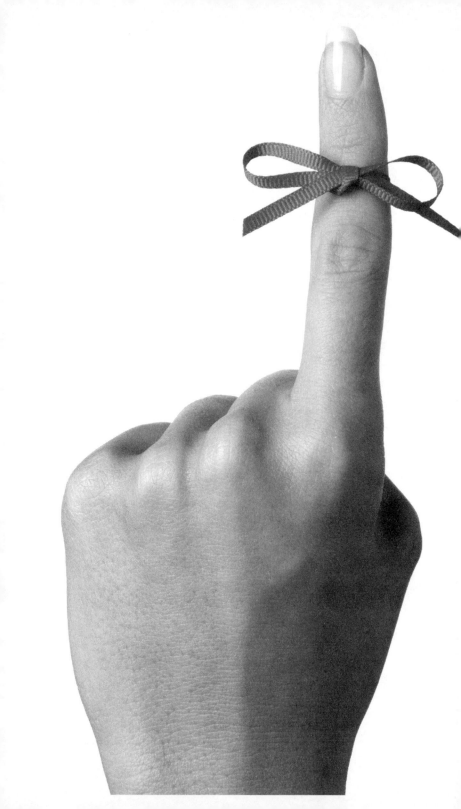

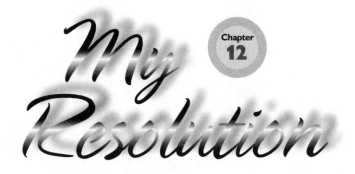

Chapter
12

Coming Full Circle

The world is round and the place which may seem like the end may also be only the beginning.

~Ivy Baker Priest

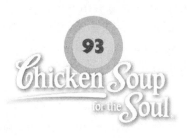

93

The Daily Resolution

The tie which links mother and child
is of such pure and immaculate strength as to be never violated.
~Washington Irving

"I don't know what I would do without you," she said, her ninety years of life reducing it to a gentle sigh.

"You'd have to live another fifty years in order for me to pay you back for all you've done for us, and maybe then it wouldn't be long enough," I answered.

I thought for a moment. Years of little league baseball, trips to the golf course, the library, the pool, the gym, and countless childhood destinations. She would take us there, gladly and often.

I've resolved to show my appreciation, although I doubt I could ever match her diligence from days long gone.

She is from the Greatest Generation. We are losing them daily, sadly. She was a Navy nurse who arrived at Pearl Harbor months after the December 7, 1941 attack. She and others like her were there to pick up the pieces and care for the wounded who would find their way there from many Pacific battles.

She has been there time and again through the years when her country and her family needed her. Patient and persevering, her work as a private duty nurse put two children through college and helped create a comfortable retirement for herself and her Navy husband. She was always there for us. The same way many of the Greatest Generation has been there when needed, always.

Today she passes time in a retirement home. She sees many of the residents struggle on a daily basis. She helps when she can. She reads them the menu at dinner, helps them at bingo, and simply offers encouragement to those who have none.

"I hate to impose on you," she whispers when it's time for her hair appointment or a trip to the grocery store.

I want her to impose because it is no imposition at all. It is a wonderful chance to help her as she helped us in our youth. Only now, I can help her in her old age.

Life for her is a day-to-day venture. Truthfully, it is for all of us as we never know what tomorrow brings to our horizon.

I have learned that from her. I've also learned from her that growing old is no easy task. She walks with a cane, slower than last year and the year before. But she keeps moving. She loves her college basketball games and eagerly goes through her morning newspaper every day.

Yes, I want to take her where she needs to go. I want to help her any way I might. This is my daily resolve.

Hopefully, there are more trips to the store, to her hairdresser, to her favorite restaurant or simply to watch golf on television at my home.

Hopefully there will be more car rides, more errands, more things she will need. One day she looked at me and declared, "I've had a good life. I'm ready to leave anytime. I don't want to live a lot longer."

"Yes you do," I responded. "I'm not ready for you to leave yet. We still have things to do."

Yes, we all do.

~Tom Edrington

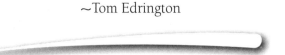

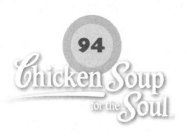

94

The Circle of Strife

When weeding, the best way to make sure you are removing a weed and not a valuable plant is to pull on it. If it comes out of the ground easily, it is a valuable plant.

~Author Unknown

My "watch" begins early each April. I stroll my yard daily like an expectant parent in search of a sign that something is about to emerge. The laws of nature tell me that the precious perennials which I planted and tended to the year before should return to me after the cold winter months have passed.

A few usually do. Others drift off into some kind of garden "black hole." And the destination of some that never reappear is usually resolved when I say to my husband, "I wonder why those Shasta Daisies that I planted by the stone wall aren't beginning to grow."

His reply is always the same.

"Oh, I thought those were weeds and pulled them."

Every spring, in spite of husband-weeding obstacles and other forces of nature, I look at my gardens through rose-colored glasses because I am certain that this will be the year my yard will take on the look of the New York Botanical Garden.

With my enthusiasm in high gear, I begin the process.

I pull weeds, mulch, and clear the dead brush from the garden beds.

I split and replant from the sprouts whose heads crown out of the ground and revel in the joy of my "free plant" bargains.

I go to the local garden store and shop 'til I drop with purchases of colorful annuals and new perennials... to replace those previously thought to be weeds.

I'm in garden nirvana!

For the next three months, I hover over the young plant life like a zealous new mother. Every evening my plant care routine prevails as I water the gardens, deadhead flowers, and spray new buds with deer spray. Each time I leave the house, I scan the horizon of my yard to make sure things are intact. It may not be the Botanical Garden, but I feel a sense of pride as I enjoy the fruits of my labor.

However, as late July approaches and the summer heat is in full force, something happens. My garden "love affair" begins to settle down. No longer is it new, fresh and exciting. The "hot" passion I once felt towards my garden goals now relates more to the sweltering summer heat.

An adventure that once offered excitement and rewards has become a chore... a chore to be done in the humidity of mid-summer!

"Maybe it will rain and I won't have to go water those stupid plants," I consider with great optimism as I turn on The Weather Channel.

By mid-August, when I walk out my front door and scan the grounds I realize my gardens have taken on a dried flower look.

Looking for excuses, I'll try to rationalize. "Didn't I see in *Better Homes and Gardens* that dried flower gardens are in this year?"

The eyesore in my yard is magnified by the display of flourishing foliage in my neighbor's yard, which closely resembles the world renowned gardens of the Palace of Versailles. Envy consumes me each time I look in their direction.

As the autumn flowers begin to appear in the garden shops, my motivation is renewed. I can visualize the displays of scruffy scarecrows nestled amongst the stacks of hay, and rich colored chrysanthemums prominently displayed in my yard. I develop a plan which allows me to salvage the shriveled plots throughout my property. And to ensure that next spring when the neighbors look in my direction they'll think they're in Holland, I add one hundred tulip bulbs to my purchase. My yard gets a respectable facelift that holds us over while the cold weather approaches.

Before I know it, another winter has passed. My seasonal "watch" resumes and, to my delight, the tulips I planted in the fall have sprouted from the ground. Yet, predictably, as I walk the property two weeks later, I see that the deer have eaten every single tulip bud off the plants, leaving only a small green sprout sticking up from the dirt!

So resumes my garden's circle of life. I accept it for what it is and continue to approach it each spring in the hopeful spirit that nature dictates. My resolve never falters and someday I hope my gardens will look like my neighbors'.

As I scan the yard, I can see that the replanted Shasta Daisies by the stone wall are beginning to emerge. Perhaps if I fence them in with yellow police tape my husband won't think they're weeds this year.

~Sharon Struth

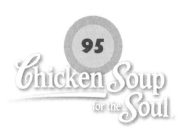

95

Strong Roots

One advantage of marriage is that, when you fall out of love with him or he falls out of love with you, it keeps you together until you fall in again.
~Judith Viorst

After thirty years we were just going through the motions. You wonder about that trite phrase, but that's really exactly what it amounted to. Every day was spelled out—what time we rose, left for work and returned, same routine—most days we even ate the same supper. Monday we had pasta, Tuesday meatloaf, and so on through the week. We found we didn't have anything new to talk about either.

"How was your day?"

"Same as usual, and yours?"

"Oh, the usual stuff."

That's what our conversations amounted to as we prepared dinner and a night of turning our brains off in front of the television. It had been different years ago. We married very young and left our native Scotland for a new country with a year-old infant. We were all we had and all we needed; we laughed and cried together and faced it all, just the three of us.

As the years went by, we enjoyed a decent level of income and settled into a comfortable lifestyle but we forgot about the simple joys of life. I remembered long ago Jim would sometimes turn up at my office unexpectedly to take me to lunch. When I saw his face, my heart would race and I would be happy for the rest of the week just thinking about that day.

Whenever we could afford to, we gave each other small gifts we knew we would enjoy, usually a new tool for Jim, and a book for me. We would treat ourselves to a special dinner now and again and relish the feeling of doing something we shouldn't, something we couldn't really afford.

The day came when we had paid for our house and put our only son through school. We could have what we wanted within reason, but we didn't buy each other little surprises anymore. We dined out each Friday evening at a modest restaurant; we were the middle-aged couple in the corner who ate quietly because we had nothing left to say to each other. Jim is a good decent man who would do anything for me, but he is a quiet man who doesn't say much and keeps his feelings to himself. Sometimes I wished he were more outgoing, more dynamic.

When we first saw our house, we had fallen in love with it. It needed a lot of work but we were happy to learn together, and we spent years making it our home. More recently, Jim had let the old house go; many small repairs didn't get done. Maybe it was a bit like our marriage; we weren't paying attention to the details. The garden didn't get the care it needed either—the trees surrounding the property badly needed trimming. One old maple's branches had grown across the driveway and were getting into the gutter and threatening to damage the roof. Every time I reminded Jim of this, he would say he would do something about it, but he never got around to it. Our next door neighbor told him the tree was leaning towards the house, but still the situation was ignored.

The inevitable happened—after a really blustery night, the tree fell on the house. Thankfully, since it was already leaning, it just sort of slipped over a bit and came to rest on the roof. It didn't do too much damage to the house, only breaking some roofing tiles. When Jim left for work the next morning, he couldn't get past the tree; as I came out the kitchen door, all I could see was Jim staring at me amidst the branches.

I looked at Jim's face, and looking back at me I saw the man I remembered from long ago. He looked like a little boy who knew he had done wrong and was waiting for the consequences. Right then, it hit me. We could keep on going as we had, or we could resolve to get what we had lost years ago. I could go on and on about how it was his fault that the tree had fallen, getting angrier and angrier every time I thought about it, or I could let it go. So I told him this would make it easier to trim the top branches and we both began to laugh.

Our neighbors were stunned to hear laughter coming through the branches that were covering the driveway. We spent the morning cutting away the lower growth so we could get to our cars, which thankfully, we had parked at the end of the driveway. Then I called the insurance company, which sent a crew to take the tree off the house and repair the roof.

That was our turning point; I resolved that things would change. Since then, we spend our supper hour talking about our day, with the television off. We go for walks in the evening through our small town. We enjoy each other's company again. I think I had shut down, and so had he; it took one of us to decide to get back what we had, for both of us to go in that direction. Life is about the small stuff; that's how we live most of our days, so we have to get the most out of each and every one of them. I had fallen in love with this man many years ago. He was still the same person I married, and the way he is, is fine by me. I just needed an old tree to reveal our strong roots.

~Christine Kettle

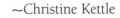

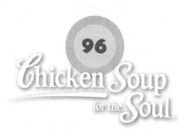

96

Brick and Stone

It takes hands to build a house, but only hearts can build a home.
~Author Unknown

When I was a boy, my mother had a small plaque that hung in the kitchen of our tiny apartment.

It read, "A house is made of brick and stone, but a home is made of love alone."

My wife and I had planned on being the typical American couple. We'd get married; work for a couple of years (to earn some stability and get to know one another), and then start our family. We had seen our friends follow this same agenda and it seemed simple enough.

We learned it was not always so simple....

Years of self-doubt, frustration, and bittersweet smiles ensued as we held the newborn babies of our closest friends, all the while agonizing over the empty place in our own home and hearts. We longed to be the parents that we KNEW God had made us to be.

Finally, after a decade of trying, and reaching the ripe old age of thirty-eight, we realized that having a baby just wasn't going to happen the "old-fashioned way."

So, we sought help.

Only to find that "help" is expensive... very expensive.

The process of IVF (in-vitro fertilization) and a subsequent pregnancy and birth would cost tens of thousands of dollars.

We had three hundred dollars in the bank.

It was a long night at the dinner table. There was anger and there were tears.

How could God put such a burning desire, such a lifelong goal to be parents in our hearts, and then make it impossible to achieve?

We didn't have tens of thousands of dollars... we didn't have one thousand dollars... but we did have our house.

Years of scrimping and saving, driving clunker cars and brown-bagging lunches had allowed us to pay off our school debts and save just enough for a down payment on a beautiful little three-bedroom, two-bath house on the outskirts of town.

Vickie and I both worked full-time, living in tiny apartments in bad neighborhoods to save money, crunching numbers until they squeaked, and jumping though every hoop imaginable for ten years to buy that house. It wasn't much, but it was ours. For a kid who'd never lived anywhere but apartment complexes, it was everything.

It was a place to have friends over, to plant our own flowers, and to paint the walls whatever shade of purple we pleased... a place of our own. It had been like a dream come true when, three years before, we'd signed papers and moved in, and now it was being made clear to us.

We could have our baby... if we gave up our home.

The market was ripe, and our agent assured us that we could get our asking price, which would leave us just enough to pay off our few remaining debts, complete the IVF process, and find a small apartment near our jobs.

We talked. We argued. We cried.

Finally, we prayed.

That's when we realized that everything we had scrimped and saved and sacrificed for had been leading to this moment. We weren't being forced out of our home, we were being given an opportunity to have the child we'd always wanted... and all we had to trade for our miracle baby was this block of brick and stone.

People all over the world suffered through childless lives, and we had been given a blank check. A check with three bedrooms, two baths, and a garage... all we had to do was sign it.

And after much soul searching, we resolved to do it.

More sacrifices were made, possessions were sold, and more tears were shed when we stood in the living room of yet another tiny two-bedroom apartment.

Then the innumerable trips to the doctor, the embarrassing medical tests, the extremely candid conversations with nurses, and the seemingly-unending "are we" or "aren't we" months of limbo, hope and heartbreak.

It's been three years since we sold our dream house, and our daughter Grace just turned one. Nothing about her addition to our family was easy—not her conception, her birth, or her first weeks at home—but she has brought light to our lives that no windows could, and colors to our world that no flowers can ever match... she is truly our miracle baby.

We're saving again for a house, and we've moved to a larger apartment, where I work part-time from home and take care of our daughter. Sometimes we talk fondly about our dream house and the memories are bittersweet.

Then baby Grace smiles, and laughs, and hugs our necks and we remember that it was just a house, brick and stone, and that this is our home... these aging rented walls, because they have been made of love.

~Perry P. Perkins

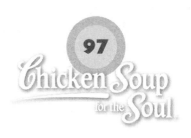

Only a Coincidence

Above all else: keep your sense of humor.
~Hugh Sidey

I must confess I was once a "re-gifter." It began forty-five years ago, long before "re-gift" became a popular word in our vocabulary after being used on an episode of *Seinfeld*.

In late October, 1963, I received a beautiful floral silk scarf for my birthday from my Aunt Zoe who lived in Florida. Even though the scarf was lovely, it really wasn't me. However, a tinge of guilt rushed through me when I considered donating the scarf to a charitable organization. Then several ideas came to mind. Surely, someone else might enjoy the scarf, and since I lived in the West, who'd be the wiser? Immediately, I set up a "re-gift drawer" in my bedroom dresser and tucked the scarf away.

Several weeks later, I wrapped the scarf elegantly and gave it to my boss at a birthday luncheon. After cake was served, I watched her open the silver gift box, slowly fold back the matching tissue and carefully lift the scarf to admire it. She smiled, raised the scarf to her chin, and brushed her cheek with the silk fabric, "It's so soft, and I adore the lovely blue and green hues. It goes so well with my navy blue suit. Thank you so much."

"I'm glad you like it," I replied, beaming, feeling smug and secretly priding myself on mastering the art of re-gifting.

Thanksgiving was only days away, and I was invited to join

my husband and staff for their annual Thanksgiving potluck. I volunteered to make a pumpkin cheesecake for the occasion.

At noon, I'd arrived with cheesecake in hand. As I stood at the front desk in the lobby, waiting for the receptionist to announce my arrival, a deliveryman handed her a birthday bouquet. "Thanks!" she squealed. "Oh, I love giant yellow mums."

After retrieving the card clipped to the arrangement, she shared the message with me—the flowers were from the office staff.

As I offered birthday wishes, she interrupted me, "They are so nice to me here," she said. "I also received a box of candy and a gorgeous silk scarf." Suddenly, she pulled the scarf from a silver box buried beneath other gift boxes stacked on the desk, and draped the delicate silk fabric around her neck.

I managed to finally utter a feeble birthday greeting, but I was stunned—it looked like the same silver box, tissue paper and floral silk scarf—could it be? Of course not, I thought, it was only a coincidence. I was grateful when my husband appeared a few seconds later and whisked me off to the potluck.

As Christmas neared, I took inventory of my re-gift drawer. I was amazed at the nice things I'd accumulated. There were two bottles of Tigress Cologne by Faberge that were all the rage, an assortment of trendy gold and silver chunky bracelets, and two simulated pearl necklaces with matching pearl drop earrings. I wrapped and adorned each re-gift with ribbons and bows, and crossed six people off my Christmas list.

Two weeks before Christmas, I attended my employer's holiday party. Since it was a small financial institution, the party was an intimate and fun-filled celebration. The highlight of the party was a white elephant gift exchange. My gift for the exchange was a fondue pot with matching tray and forks. The gifts ranged from exquisite to outlandish—the great thing about this type of gift exchange was the stealing and the trading.

After dinner we all pulled a number from a festive green basket. "Let the game begin!" my boss shouted. Since I drew number one, I was the first to choose a gift. I admired the shiny foil holly wrapping paper, then untied the red ribbons and ripped open the package. I was dumbstruck... instantly... I recognized the silver gift box tied with the silver sequined ribbon. For a moment, I was engulfed with a glimmer of hope. Surely, it was only a coincidence... but as I unfolded the tissue paper, there was no mistaking the blue and green floral silk scarf tucked inside.

The fondue set I'd brought was the most popular item stolen and traded that evening. But to my dismay, no one wanted to trade or steal the scarf. At the end of the evening, I smiled, wrapped the exquisite scarf around my neck, and made a silent vow to make a New Year's resolution not to re-gift ever again.

The champagne flowed freely at our neighborhood New Year's Eve party. At the stroke of midnight, I toasted the New Year with my husband and four of our closest friends. Immediately, everyone took turns stating their New Year's resolutions. I waited until last... I just couldn't tell them about the scarf incident... I took a deep breath, lifted my glass, glanced around the room, and declared, "I don't believe in making New Year's resolutions. Besides, who keeps resolutions anyway? Not me."

Laughter ensued, as we raised our glasses and sang "Auld Lang Syne."

I have never told a soul... until now... that I made that resolution to never re-gift again. Actually, it is the only New Year's resolution I have ever kept.

~Georgia A. Hubley

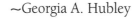

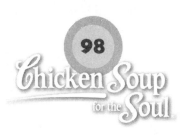

98

The Flames of Forgiveness

Forgive all who have offended you, not for them, but for yourself.
~Harriet Nelson

M y father passed away in a nursing home on a September day. He lived in the Northeast and I lived in the South. He had been an extremely proud man who kept his family under his thumb with his passionate religious beliefs and his stern disciplinary actions.

I never remembered my father telling me he loved me, and upon hearing of his death, I did not feel the need to cry. I struggled with my lack of remorseful feelings over his passing, knowing it was not healthy for me to avoid grieving.

On Christmas Day of that year, I was reflecting on as many good memories of my father as I could. I decided I would make it my New Year's resolution to work out my feelings and become "unstuck," so I sat down and wrote my father a letter.

Dear Daddy,

I remembered something today. I remembered when I was about two or three years old. Mom carried me into your bedroom right before bedtime and you sang "Now I Lay Me down To Sleep" to me, and I remember your voice like it was just yesterday. You had a lovely baritone voice. I remember the warmth of you lying next to me and how special I felt at that moment. Then Mom appeared and carried me off to my own bed to tuck me in.

I remembered times when I would sit out on the porch with you and watch an approaching thunderstorm, and you would tell me the scientific facts behind lightning and thunder. I thought you knew everything.

In early spring, you would make me work in the vegetable garden and plant seeds with you. Many times I'd rather be doing other things, but when the plants started to rise out of the soil, I was amazed.

I remember you taking my two brothers and me on trips to a creek out in the country on summer days. We would pile out of the car and go walking along the creek, picking wildflowers to take home to Mother. I want to thank you for giving me an appreciation of nature and science and of God's beautiful creation, Earth.

I want to thank you for making us take part in "family worship" every evening after dinner, even though, as a growing child, I would rather have been out playing with my friends. I remember the Bible stories, and the Golden Rule on how to treat others, and I learned how to appreciate music in my life from the hymns we sang. I also learned to harmonize with my sisters. I don't know what I would do without music in my life today.

And most of all, I want to forgive you. I forgive you for not being able to tell me that I was a special little girl and that you loved me. I longed for your spoken affection. But I realize that something in your own upbringing would not allow you to express your feelings verbally. I realize that you did the best that you could with what you knew.

I signed the letter, folded it, and put it in my grandmother's cedar chest to join the many other cards and letters from family and loved ones that I cherished. But somehow, it had not brought the closure that I desired.

A week later, on New Year's Eve, I remembered the letter to my father. I retrieved it from the cedar chest and took it outside to the backyard. Then I built a small fire and dropped the letter into the flames and watched it burn.

As I thanked my father for giving me life, the tears came. I released all the pent-up grief and whispered, "You were my father... and I love you."

~Beverly Walker

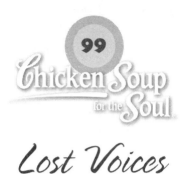

99

Lost Voices

Letters are among the most significant memorial
a person can leave behind them.
~Johann Wolfgang von Goethe

Sometimes the best resolutions involve a sincere attempt to do something nice for a stranger when no one is looking. That is what my wife, Barbara, resolved to do with a forgotten box from a dusty attic.

"You might be interested in these."

My father-in-law stood holding an old cardboard box. It smelled of dust and paper too long without air.

"What is it?" I asked, taking the box.

"Some letters and other things. I thought you might be interested."

He had found the box in the attic of an old, vacant house in Highland Park, an exclusive neighborhood just north of Dallas. It was being renovated. He had been running air-conditioning ducts in the attic.

"I talked to the real estate agent," he said. "He has no idea who they belong to. Looks like the box has been up in that attic for years."

I set the box down and opened it. A lot of letters. Underneath the envelopes, a stack of black composition books. The first was dated across the top in long hand. It was fifty years old.

I took them home. So began my introduction to the Mathis family of Dallas. The letters spanned from the twenties to the fifties. Most were from Mr. Mathis to his wife. He traveled a lot. Elegant prose graced hotel stationery from all across Texas. He wrote of loneliness and love, asked about his two sons, and spoke of their future. There were letters from Jim and Jack, the sons, describing college and life in general. Both boys' prose was as articulate as the parents', expressing themselves in a manner that could only be described as word craft. The art of letters. The lost voice.

Just as engrossing were the notebooks. Mrs. Mathis' diaries spanned decades, gorgeously describing everyday life. She wrote of life in the 1920s and '30s in Dallas. The streetcars. The shops. The grand show houses along Elm and Commerce. The cost of house-wares, the minute details of her garden. Thoughts of the boys as they grew up. Idle chatter, eloquently expressed. Deep feelings about her husband. Questions. All those years, quiet in the box, in the attic of an old house. Lost.

I tried half-heartedly to find the family. No related Mathis in Dallas. I gave up, finally putting the books and letters away. For close to twenty years, I kept them in a black footlocker. During that period, I must have moved ten times, was divorced, changed jobs and married again. The letters and diaries remained in the footlocker. Occasionally, usually during a move, I would pop open the lid again and browse through them, still charmed by the words that flowed from their pens. I would revisit the Mathis family for a few minutes, and then put them away.

It was during a re-organization of our college-bound son's room that my wife and I once again stumbled over the footlocker. Again we perused. Again we marveled. Yet this time, it stayed out of the closet.

Barbara, my wife, was a teacher. It was summer. Finally, she had more than two minutes a day to relax. Between catching up on a thousand chores and raising our youngest, she read the diaries and letters. The love between sons and parents jumped off the pages, as alive as the day the elaborately swirled letters were first put to paper.

"Someone would want these," she said, one afternoon, a letter in her hand. "The boys would. I am going to look for them."

"Fine," I said. It was 1992. "I tried once. Some of that stuff is older than you and I put together. You'll be wasting your time."

What I failed to consider is that Barbara never wastes time. She did the normal things. Called all the Mathis listings in the phone book. Reread the diaries. Searched for clues in the letters. One was they had relatives in Tyler, so she looked there. No luck.

Then one day while skimming one of the diaries, she came across a folded paper in the back of the book. It was the Highland Park High School 1937 "Graduation and Commencement" program. Jack's program. That gave her an idea. She reached the high school's alumni association. Jack Mathis lived in New Jersey. She called him. Yes, he had a brother named Jim. Yes, he once lived in Dallas on Victor.

Bingo. She had found them. Neither parent was alive. Jim lived in Wisconsin. The Mathis brothers were now in their sixties. Over the years, they had wondered about the diaries, knew their mother kept them the entirety of their childhoods and beyond, but had long ago given up hope of ever finding them.

So my wife removed the letters and the composition books from the black footlocker and placed them in a sturdy cardboard box. There were children and grandchildren waiting in New Jersey and Wisconsin for the beautiful words formed by the hearts of their grandparents. She mailed the box.

At Christmas time, a gift arrived from Jack. With it came a gracious letter, the familiar prose moving across the page like a melody. It ended, "Words cannot express our gratitude."

I thought about that. Maybe not. Yet for one family, words certainly expressed everything. Words no longer silent. Voices found.

~James Blackshear

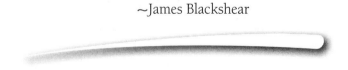

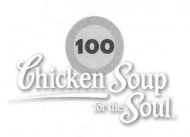

Gifts of Resolve

The only true gift you can give is a portion of thyself.
~Ralph Waldo Emerson

The bills were coming in, and just as I had done during the previous thirty-six years of our married life, I put them in a box. After separating them by order of urgency, I made a mental note of anything that needed immediate attention. The only difference now was they all seemed to have the word "urgent" stamped on them. Since late spring, we had been feeling the effects of the economy, but never before had our comfortable way of life felt so uncomfortable!

We had never really lived beyond our means. And now with our children grown and married, we were looking forward to retirement in a few years and were making decisions about where to live. We had planned to take some mini-vacations to various places we might enjoy living, to check them out. Our home was worth much more than what we had paid for it ten years ago, and we continued to make improvements, waiting for just the right time to place it on the market.

My husband is a builder, but in the worsening economy the demand for construction diminished. A couple who had planned to have my husband build a home for them seemed to focus on the economy a bit more, and other scheduled jobs with clients were placed on hold as well. In the meantime, many builders left the Island, and my husband picked up renovation work wherever he could. It all seemed so unbelievable. The Island where we lived had been thriving. People were building and times were good; and suddenly it came to a screeching halt.

I wanted to go back to work, but a back injury limited what I was able to do, and so I did what I knew best. I resolved to economize. I reviewed our situation; I got rid of my own cell phone and made some changes to our phone/cable/TV plan. When our car lease was up, I didn't renew it. I rationalized that now we would save the lease payment and the insurance premium, and with gas prices so high we could save even more.

I looked for other ways to cut back. I enjoyed making soups and having fresh veggie dinners over the summer and fall. I often made breakfast into a dinner meal and I watched our grocery purchases. Very few meals were eaten out. It all added up.

Purchasing birthday gifts for family and friends has always been special for me. I enjoy taking the time to think about the birthday person and finding just the right gift. But with my resolve to economize, I knew there would have to be some changes made in my gift buying routine. I came up with a plan.

I recalled my grandmother giving various items to family members when she moved out of her big home and downsized. Those gifts were always very special to me. I looked at my own cups and saucer collection; some miniature sizes had been used for storybook teas with area children when we first had moved to the Island; so I chose a lovely pink floral English bone china design that would be just perfect for our eight-year-old granddaughter. She loved tea parties. I knew the other grandchildren's likes and dislikes and I would give them something that I had enjoyed in order to continue the tradition that my grandmother had started. For birthdays and other holidays, each person would get a gift of love, an item that I had cherished.

With the possibility of moving, I also resolved to de-clutter a bit. Items that I didn't want to move, and other things that I knew our children didn't want, went to an area consignment shop. We would have less to pack when and if the time came to actually make the move, and get some return on our initial investment to boot!

I have faith in knowing the Lord is directing our entire situation, and that our great nation will once again see prosperity. So many are going through so much at this time, and I'm well aware that our own situation could be much worse. I believe people who hold onto hope and can cut back will realize we are still fortunate to be living in the greatest land on earth, and we are blessed by how much we truly have.

~Diane Dean White

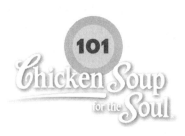

Let's Celebrate the Old

Old wood best to burn, old wine to drink, old friends to trust,
and old authors to read.
~Quoted by Francis Bacon

It used to be that every time the new year rolled around, I marched headlong into it, looking forward to the opportunity to try out a new notion. Go with a bolder color in the kitchen. Find a new hair-do. Learn a new skill.

I hate to sound disagreeable, and maybe my age is showing, but these days I am finding more and more comfort in the "oldness" of things.

Here are a few old things that should be celebrated every new year:

Old Shoes—They may not look debonair, but they feel terrific. Instead of pinching that pesky corn on your little toe, or squeezing that bunion on your right foot, old shoes have made the necessary adjustments—lifting a bit here, stretching a bit there—making sure your aging feet have little to complain about.

Old Folks—We live in a society where young people are put on a pedestal and idolized, while old folks are forgotten. But if you want to draw from a well of knowledge and wisdom, inquire of the elderly. Not only do their stories entertain, but their advice can keep you from making mistakes of your own and help steer you in the right direction.

Old Friends—I enjoy making new friends, but old friends who

have shared my pain and sorrow, celebrated my joys, and remained steadfast when trouble came knocking; they are the ones I will celebrate most in the New Year.

Old Clothes—I enjoy a new outfit as much as the next woman, but please don't ask me to give up my old bathrobe, my old sweater, or that old T-shirt that wears like a cloud.

Old Stuff—When looking at the medley of things I have collected through the years, I am struck by the thought that my home is mostly filled with objects that have been cast out by others. I suppose I should feel a bit miffed about that, but, oddly enough, I find solace in being surrounded by old things. There's nothing new that can compare to old books, old quilts, old photographs, old letters, old recipes, old rocking chairs, and old toys.

Old Husbands—My husband and I just celebrated twenty-eight years of marriage. Together, we have lived through serious illnesses and a host of major surgeries. We've nursed broken ankles, broken toes, broken shoulders, and broken hearts. We've engaged in bitter quarrels, and endured excruciating marriage counseling. There were times when it would have been so much easier to walk away—and times when we almost did. But we stayed committed to our wedding vows, and I'm very glad that we did, because I can't imagine growing old with anyone else.

Old Truths—like those found in the stirring words of our revered president Abraham Lincoln: "It is the duty of nations, as well as of men, to own their dependence upon the overruling power of God and to recognize the sublime truth announced in the Holy Scriptures and proven by all history, that those nations only are blessed whose God is the Lord."

Old Glory—Every time I see the American flag waving in the breeze, I remember that freedom isn't free, and never has been. I'm reminded of the words of John Quincy Adams: "Posterity—you will never know how much it has cost my generation to preserve your freedom. I hope you will make good use of it."

Maybe next January I'll be in the mood to turn over a new leaf, tackle a new project, or celebrate a new trend. But for now, I am perfectly content with the old.

~Dayle Allen Shockley

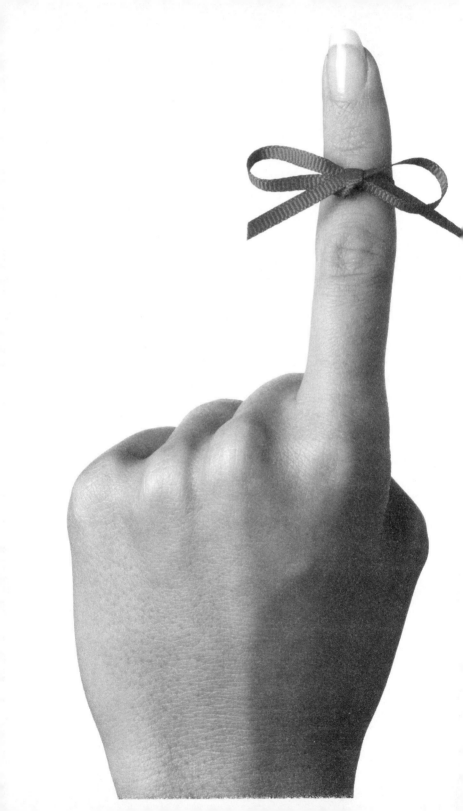

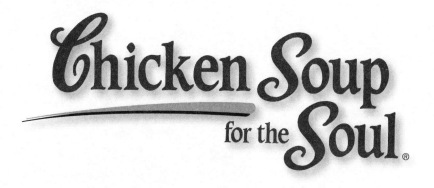

Meet Our Contributors!
About the Authors
Acknowledgments

Chicken Soup for the Soul

Meet Our Contributors!

Charles Baker, once afraid to submit work like most of his students, is now The Writing Coach, and has hundreds of published works including poetry, magazine articles, and fiction and nonfiction books. His greatest writing thrill though is seeing his students and his clients publish. Contact him at mywritingstuff@yahoo.com.

Carol Band is a mother of three who chronicles life in the trenches of suburbia. Visit her website www.carolband.com or e-mail her at carol@carolband.com.

Deborah Batt is a Social Worker currently working in the Adoption Department of the Children's Aid Society. She enjoys traveling and working with children and aspires to work overseas in an orphanage. She has completed her first novel and is writing a second, hoping to inspire others through her words.

Joan McClure Beck has a bachelors and a master's degree. Retired as an elementary school reading specialist, she now teaches adult basic education.

Alexandra Mochary Bergstein was a corporate attorney but now dedicates herself to raising three children and learning about all things "Green." A graduate of Wesleyan University and University of Chicago Law School, she practiced law at the firm of Skadden, Arps. She and her family live happily in Greenwich, CT.

James Blackshear retired from Lincoln Property Company in 2006, returned to school and received a Masters in history from Texas A&M Commerce in 2008. He is currently writing a history of New Mexico land grants. He and his wife, Barbara, split time between New Mexico and Texas.

Lil Blosfield has enjoyed writing for over thirty years and recently won first prize in the *Chicken Soup for the American Idol Soul* contest. She works as CFO for Child and Adolescent Behavioral Health in Canton, Ohio. She enjoys playing the piano and spending time with her family and friends.

Cynthia Briggs celebrates her love of cooking and writing through her nostalgic cookbook, *Pork Chops & Applesauce* and her apple dessert cookbook titled *Sweet Apple Temptations*. She is currently writing *Pork Chops & Applesauce, Second Helping* and *Sassy Starters*. Contact Cynthia through her website, www.porkchopsandapplesauce.net.

Linda Butler lives in the beautiful mountains of Utah where she enjoys raising her children and assorted critters. She likes to garden, hike, read, and discover new joys in the world around her. Still quiet, but no longer shy, Linda works as a correspondent for a weekly community newspaper.

Kristine Byron is an interior decorator, writer of children's stories and is in the process of writing her first cookbook. She is looking to have her stories illustrated and published. Kristine enjoys cooking, entertaining and spending time with her grandchildren. You can reach her at rbyron14@aol.com.

Molly Cadigan is the Editor of a small news magazine in Bobcaygeon, Ontario. She is the author of a humorous column based on her experiences in motherhood, and aspires to write fiction for children and young women.

Jeri Chrysong writes to share her journey into wellness. Her writings have appeared in *Chicken Soup for the Soul* and other inspirational books. She resides in Huntington Beach, CA, with two spoiled pugs.

Her hobbies include family, photography, writing, and annual sojourns to Hawaii. Jeri. Contact her via e-mail at jchrysong@aol.com.

Harriet Cooper is a freelance writer living in Toronto, Canada. She is a frequent contributor to *Chicken Soup for the Soul* and often writes about health, diet, and family. When not writing for magazines, newspapers, newsletters, and anthologies, she continues to exercise, eat healthy, and curb her enthusiasm for junk food.

Janet M. Cromer, RN, MA is a Psychotherapist and award-winning freelance writer in Jamaica Plain, MA. Janet is completing her memoir book, *Professor Cromer Learns to Read—A Couple's New Life after Brain Injury*. Janet enjoys hiking, kayaking, gardening, reading, and participating in writing classes of all kinds.

Barbara Curtis lives with her husband Tripp and the last five of their twelve children in Bluemont, VA. Barbara is also a prolific writer with nine books and 900+ articles to her credit. She blogs daily at www.MommyLife.net.

Priscilla Dann-Courtney is a writer and clinical psychologist in Boulder, CO. where she lives with her husband and three children. She is an avid runner and finds peace of mind through yoga and meditation. She is a newspaper columnist and is currently working on a book of her essays.

Mary Hay Davis is a freelance writer living in southern California with her husband and two teenage sons. Before her serendipitous transformation into a professional writer, she worked previously as a police dispatcher—an occupation rich in tales of the foibles and frailties of the human condition. Contact Mary at: writeforyou@cox.net.

Mary J. Davis has sold more than 1,000 articles, many co-written with her husband, Larry, and more than fifty books. She has contributed to several *Chicken Soup for the Soul* books and other anthologies.

She and Larry live in Montrose, IA, and have three grown children and eight grandchildren.

Michele Ivy Davis is a freelance writer whose stories and articles have appeared in a variety of magazines and anthologies as well as in newspapers and law enforcement publications. Her young adult novel, *Evangeline Brown and the Cadillac Motel* has won national and international awards. Learn more at www.MicheleIvyDavis.com.

Laura Dean is a stay-at-home mom of two adorable boys. This is her first contribution to *Chicken Soup for the Soul*. Laura cares deeply about the environment and continues to teach her children the importance of taking care of those less fortunate.

Rebecca Degtjarjov attended Elgin Community College, earning a place in the PTK Honors Society before heading off to explore the world. With her newfound energy she's backpacked across Mexico, England, and France. She now resides in Northern California with her husband and Anatolian Shepherd. Please e-mail her at writer_madness@yahoo.com.

Steve Delmonte left advertising after five years, and started drawing cartoons and doing humorous illustrations for magazines, ad agencies and book publishers. His work has appeared in *Barron's, Woman's World, First For Women, Nelson, Readers Digest, Scholastic, Field & Stream* and *National Enquirer*. Reach him at steve@stevedelmontestudio.com.

Tom Edrington lives in Tampa, Florida. He is a graduate of East Carolina University and a former sports writer for the Tampa Tribune. Tom enjoys spending time with his wife Micki and Mya, their Min-Pin. He writes for examiner.com and is available for quality free lance assignment. Please e-mail him at flrealtyinc@aol.com.

HJ Eggers recently returned from the Maui Writers Retreat and attended classes taught by John Lescroart. She's overjoyed to announce her inaugural book, *The Prodigal Wife*. A chastened woman seeks reconciliation with her family, but stumbles into a storm. Watch for it in 2009. E-mail her at hjs01234@aol.com.

Terri Elders lives near Colville, WA, with husband, Ken Wilson. *My Resolution* will be her fifth *Chicken Soup for the Soul* book. She also has stories in the upcoming *A Cup of Comfort* books for young mothers and for adoptive families, and *My Dad is My Hero*. Write her at telders@hotmail.com.

Britteny Elrick attended Regents College in London, England, where she began her freelance writing career. She is a business owner and aspiring author of non-fiction books. Britteny cannot resist: a sense of humor, anything Italian, confidence, or sweatpants. Or cupcakes. You can stalk her at www.wordsbybrit.com.

Judy Epstein is the creator of an award-winning column, "A Look On the Light Side." In a previous life, she wrote and produced for Public Television. She lives with her husband, two sons, and many excellent resolutions on Long Island, New York. Please visit or e-mail her at alookonthelightside.com.

Melissa Face received her Bachelor of Arts from Coastal Carolina University and her Master of Human Resources from Webster University. She graduated with honors in 2005. Melissa currently works as an English teacher at a private school and writes on a freelance basis. Please e-mail her at writermsface@yahoo.com.

For three decades, **Sally Friedman** of Moorestown, New Jersey, has been chronicling her life for various publications including *The New York Times, Ladies' Home Journal, Family Circle* and regional newspapers and magazines. She writes about her life as a wife, mother, grandmother and observer. Contact Sally via e-mail at pinegander@aol.com.

Kimberlee Garrett is the quintessential minivan driving, PTA President, soccer mom of three wonderful children. Being a wife and mother is her dream, but when she does have a minute to herself, she rides her bike and pretends she's the first woman to win the Tour de France!

Debbie Gill lives in Brooklin, Ontario and is a mother of five who works as a supply secretary for the local school board. A community writer and reporter for the town's news publication, she is a history buff who loves to travel. Please e-mail her at debbie.gill@rogers.com.

Annita Hammonds received her Bachelor of Arts from the University of Georgia in 1996. She lives in Jonesboro, GA with her husband Albert, and her two sons, Xavier and Cameron. When not writing, Annita enjoys singing and teaching elementary school.

Emily Sue Harvey writes to make a difference. Her upbeat stories appear in numerous anthologies including *Chicken Soup for the Soul, Chocolate for Women*, and ladies' magazines. Her mainstream novel, *Song of Renewal*, published by Story Plant, will be released Spring, 2009. Emily Sue hosts www.revivalstories.com, or contact her at emilysue1@aol.com.

Sonja Herbert is the author of an award-winning, as yet unpublished novel about her mother surviving the Holocaust in a circus, and of many other true stories. Sonja currently lives in Germany, where she is doing research and getting re-acquainted with her mother and siblings. Her website is germanwriter.com.

Freelance writer and editor **Mandy Houk** teaches creative writing in Colorado Springs where she lives with her husband, Pete, and their two daughters. Mandy was born in Georgia and returned to her southern roots when writing her first novel (currently under review by agents). www.mandyhouk.com.

Georgia A. Hubley retired after twenty years in financial management to write full time. She's a frequent contributor to the *Chicken Soup for* *the Soul Series, Christian Science Monitor* and numerous other magazines, newspapers and anthologies. She resides with her husband of thirty years in Henderson, Nevada. Contact her at a geohub@aol.com.

Rebecca Jay writes from the heartland of Kansas where she enjoys the changing seasons. She works for a nonprofit organization and also teaches English and Bible to Chinese friends. Rebecca has one grown son and an elderly cat.

Vickey Kalambakal, freelance writer, went back to school in her forties to earn a masters degree in history. Her grandsons think it's cool to see her name in magazines and books, especially when she writes about Julius Caesar and his Roman legions. Her e-mail address is Vickey@Kalambakal.com.

Karen Kelly's career currently encompasses the entire trinity of media: radio, TV and print. Her weekly column, "Karen's Korner" expresses her many interests and beliefs. Karen lives in Ohio with her husband and two dogs. She is currently working on two fiction books. Please e-mail Karen at: karenkellybrown@aol.com.

Born in Glasgow, Scotland, **Christine Kettle** lives in a small village in Southern Ontario. After a long corporate career, Christine is now enjoying new challenges, the best of which is writing.

Walt Klis was born a natural gag cartoonist, won first prize in Mason Mint's cartoon contest in 1950 with over ten thousand entries at age six. He currently has a full color page in *Games* magazine called "Punchlines."

Mimi Greenwood Knight is a freelance writer and mother of four living in South Louisiana with her husband, David, and far too many animals. She is blessed to have stories in over a dozen *Chicken Soup for the Soul* books as well as national parenting magazine and Christian magazines, anthologies, devotionals and websites.

Jeannie Lancaster lives in Loveland, Colorado. She returned to school at a "mature" age and received her BA in Communication. Following graduation, she worked in health care public relations for several years. As a freelance writer, she now explores her love of writing and words through a variety of media.

Jennifer Lawler is a writer in the Midwest, focusing on martial arts and empowerment issues. Her website is www.jenniferlawler.com.

Tim Martin is the author of four books and seven screenplays. His script *Fast Pitch* is currently in preproduction at Promenade Pictures. He has two children's novels, *Scout's Oaf*(Cedar Grove Books) and *Fast Pitch* (Blitz Publishing), scheduled for publication in 2009. Tim can be reached at tmartin@northcoast.com.

Tina Wagner Mattern is a happily married Portland Oregon writer/ hairstylist/file clerk who believes that a good sense of humor is a wonderful gift from God, paving the way for a peaceful, joyful life. Tina was last published in *Chicken Soup for the Breast Cancer Survivor's Soul*. E-mail her at tinamattern@earthlink.net.

Dahlynn McKowen has created many titles for the *Chicken Soup for the Soul* series, including *Chicken Soup for the Soul in Menopause* and *Chicken Soup for the Entrepreneur's Soul*. She and Ken own Publishing Syndicate, offering on-line writing/publishing tips for anthologies such as *Chicken Soup for the Soul*. Get their free newsletter at www.PublishingSyndicate.com.

Ken McKowen has created many titles for *Chicken Soup for the Soul*. An owner of Publishing Syndicate (www.PublishingSyndicate.com), an on-line business that offers writing/publishing tips, Ken's also developing www.PlacesToDiscover.com. This site offers stories/photos from all over the world for editors, travel and real estate agents, plus travel info for tourists.

Stacy Murphy received her Bachelor of Science from Texas A&M University in 1988. She has spent the last twenty years navigating the testosterone-laden waters of the meat industry. She now lives in East Texas and writes part-time about whatever moves her. Stacy loves animals, movies and rocking chairs.

Mark Musolf grew up in Illinois and now lives in Minnesota. He enjoys spending time with his family and making stained glass.

Linda Sue O'Connell is happiest surrounded by children. Her grand-children and students have given her many laugh lines over the years. Linda is a widely-published writer; her work has appeared in several *Chicken Soup for the Soul* books and others. She and her husband Bill, enjoy long walks on the beach. Contact her at billin7@juno.com.

Gina Otto wrote the award-winning children's book, *Cassandra's Angel*. After walking away from a twelve-year career in Hollywood, Gina has been working for more than a decade with girls and women on self-esteem and media consciousness. Gina's work invites girls and women to find their light within. Please visit her at www.CassandrasAngel.com.

Mark Parisi's "off the mark" comic, syndicated since 1987, is distributed by United Media. Mark's humor also graces greeting cards, T-shirts, calendars, magazines, newsletters and books. Check out: offthemark.com. Lynn is his wife/business partner. Their daughter, Jen, contributes inspiration (as do three cats).

Kathleen Partak lives in Northern California with her husband Dave and their young son Mason. Besides penning a weekly e-mail column for the past nine years, Kathleen also writes for local publications on topics including real estate mortgages, today's technology, and military life (Dave is a National Guard member). kdpartak@yahoo.com.

Ava Pennington is a freelance writer, speaker, and Bible teacher, with an MBA from St. John's University and a Bible Studies Certificate from

Moody Bible Institute. She has published national magazine articles and contributed stories to ten *Chicken Soup for the Soul* books and three *Cup of Comfort* books. Learn more at www.avawrites.com.

Saralee Perel is an award-winning nationally syndicated columnist and novelist. She is proud to be a multiple contributor to *Chicken Soup for the Soul*. Her novel, *Raw Nerves*, received the BookSense honor. Please visit her website at: www.saraleeperel.com. Saralee welcomes e-mails at sperel@saraleeperel.com.

Christian author **Perry P. Perkins** was born and raised in Oregon. His novels include *Just Past Oysterville*, and *Shoalwater Voices*. Perry is a student of Jerry B. Jenkins Christian Writer's Guild and a frequent contributor to the *Chicken Soup for the Soul* anthologies. Perry's work can be found online at www.perryperkinsbooks.com.

Stephanie Piro lives in New Hampshire with her husband and three cats. She is one of King Features' "Six Chix" (she is the Saturday chick!). Her single panel, "Fair Game," appears in newspapers and on her website: www.stephaniepiro.com. She also designs gift items for her company Strip T's. Contact her via e-mail at stephaniepiro@verizon.

Helen Polaski has authored hundreds of short stories and articles. She is an anthology editor for *Adams Media* and has compiled and edited eight books to date, including an anthology titled *Christmas through a Child's Eyes*. Helen and her husband spend quality time together making teensy-weensy elf doors, fairy doors and pixie doors. See www.theelfdoor.com.

Valerie Porter is a freelance writer specializing in travel, animals and the metaphysical/spiritual world. She shares her life with a wonderful husband, Kenny, her Maltese, Daphne, and her English Cocker Spaniel, David.

Joe Rector is a freelance writer who writes columns for two local newspapers and other magazines. He has made other contributions to *Chicken Soup for the Soul* books. Joe has retired from teaching high school English after thirty years. He has created a website for teachers, www.teachertales.net and a blog at www.thecommonisspectacular.com. Please e-mail Joe at joeerector@comcast.com.

Startled to discover her childhood toys in an antique mart, **Carol McAdoo Rehme** giggled—and wrote about it. Freelance editor, author, and ghostwriter, she publishes prolifically in the inspirational market and is coauthor of seven books. Carol's latest project was *Chicken Soup for the Soul: Empty Nesters*, 2008. Contact: carol@rehme.com; www.rehme.com.

Bruce Robinson is an award-winning internationally published cartoonist whose work has appeared in numerous periodicals including *The National Enquirer, The Saturday Evening Post, Woman's World, The Sun, First, Highlights*, and many others. He is also the author of the cartoon book *Good Medicine*. Contact him via e-mail at cartoonsbybrucerobinson@hotmail.com.

Sallie A. Rodman is an award-winning author whose stories have appeared in over twenty *Chicken Soup for the Soul* books. She also writes for magazines and *The Orange County Register*. She is currently working on her life story to help others, entitled, *Panic Demons...* what else? Reach her at sa.rodman@verizon.net.

Maureen Rogers is a transplanted Canadian living in the Seattle, Washington area. Her writing projects include fiction, poetry and essays. She has been published online, in newspapers, anthologies and in *Chicken Soup for the Coffee Lover's Soul*. She can be reached via e-mail at morogers@gmail.com.

Linda Ruddy finds humor in everyday events. She is channeling her creative energy into writing after much encouragement from friends. Living on Lake Ontario, she is in the throes of new home construction.

If she retains her sanity, the project should provide plenty of story material. E-mail her at lsruddy@gmail.com.

Ashley Sanders is a wife and mother, living in Kentucky. She enjoys crafting, traveling, writing, and working with children. You can find more of her writing and adventures at www.bosssanders.com and www.firstimpressionsbaby.com/blog.

Theresa Sanders has four grown children, her greatest joy and accomplishment. She graduated with honors from the University of Maryland, worked for years as a technical writer, and has published in trade journals. She lives with her husband near St. Louis, and is thrilled to be featured in *Chicken Soup for the Soul: My Resolution.*

Harriet May Savitz, a prolific contributor to *Chicken Soup for the Soul*, is the author of twenty-six books, including *Run Don't Walk*, an ABC Afterschool Special produced by Henry Winkler, and a new book, *The Gifts Animals Can Give*. Several of her books can be found at www. iUniverse.com, www.harrietmaysavitz.com or at www.authorhouse. com. Contact: greetingsfromasburypark@verizon.net.

Al Serradell is a recovering Public Relations executive who works as a Compliance Officer for the State of Oklahoma and continues to write as the spirit allows.

Joyce Newman Scott worked as a flight attendant for Eastern Airlines while pursuing an acting career. She started college in her mid-fifties and studies at the University of Miami. She is currently working on a memoir, a television script, and a feature film. Please contact her at jnewmansco@aol.com.

Dayle Allen Shockley is an award-winning writer whose by-line has appeared in dozens of publications. She is the author of three books and a contributor to many other works, including the *Chicken Soup for the Soul* series. E-mail her at dayle@dayleshockley.com.

Deborah Shouse is a speaker, writer and editor. Her writing has appeared in *Reader's Digest, Newsweek* and *Spirituality & Health.* She is donating all proceeds from her book *Love in the Land of Dementia: Finding Hope in the Caregiver's Journey* to Alzheimer's programs and research. Visit her website at www.thecreativityconnection.com.

Maggie Lamond Simone is an award-winning writer and graduate of William Smith College and the S.I. Newhouse School of Communications. Her essays have appeared in *Misadventures of Moms* and *Disasters of Dads* and *Hello, Goodbye,* as well as *Cosmopolitan.* She is the author of two children's books and an upcoming memoir.

Gail Small is a Fulbright Memorial Scholar and a People to People Ambassador. She is in Who's Who Among America's Universities and Who's Who Among America's Teachers. Travel is her passion and she has visited all seven continents! E-mail this educator, consultant, and motivational speaker at JoyforGail@aol.com. Learn more about this five-time published author at www.GailSmall.com.

Mary Z. Smith is a regular contributor to *Angels on Earth* Magazine and *Guideposts Magazine.* She resides in Richmond, VA with her husband Barry. They have four grown children, two biological and two adopted. Mary loves writing for the Lord, walking, and gardening. Please e-mail her at stillbrook@comcast.net.

Patricia Smith is a Mt. View-based freelance writer. Moose 'O My Heart is her third published *Chicken Soup for the Soul* story.

Sarah Jo Smith received a Bachelor of Arts in English Literature and holds a Master of Education from Santa Clara University. She taught middle and high school English, and classic literature through her community's Adult Education Department. She is currently completing her first novel. She lives in Los Gatos, California.

Laurie Sontag is a California writer who wishes motherhood had come with instructions. She writes a weekly column for the *Gilroy Dispatch*. You can see her work at www.lauriesontag.com or on her blog at www.manicmotherhood.com.

Sharon Struth is a freelance writer who lives in Bethel, Connecticut with her two teenage daughters, two dogs and husband of twenty years. Her work can also be seen in *Sasee* Magazine and the soon to be released *A Cup of Comfort for New Mothers*.

Nancy Sullivan holds multiple degrees and has written extensively over her career in the disability arena. She just completed a mystery novel with plans to write many more. She volunteers in animal rescue and is a Reiki Master Teacher and certified Laughter Yoga leader. Contact her at nancy.writes@sbcglobal.net.

Glorianne Swenson is a Minnesota-based published freelance writer and small business owner of gloribks. Her genre includes creative non-fiction memoirs, devotionals, poetry, and children's picture book manuscripts. She is a wife, mother, and grandmother, and enjoys singing, piano, genealogy and antiquing. She may be e-mailed at gloribks@charter.net.

B.J. Taylor works from home with her husband and loves every minute of it. She is an award-winning author whose work has appeared in *Guideposts*, many *Chicken Soup for the Soul* books, and numerous magazines and newspapers. She has a wonderful husband, four children and two adorable grandsons. You can reach B.J. at www.clik.to/bjtaylor.

Karen Theis, married thirty-five years, mother to Holly and William, is a nine-year breast cancer survivor. The Founder and President of cancer support group The Glow Girls, she was awarded the True Valley Hero Award and Community Builders Award. Her stories appear in *Chicken Soup for the Breast Cancer Survivor's Soul* and *Chicken Soup for the Beach Lover's Soul*.

Cristy Trandahl is a former teacher and writer for the nation's leading student progress monitoring company. Today she works as a freelance writer while raising her children. Visit www.cristytrandahl.com for more.

Donna L. Turello earned a Master's in English Lit. A member of Romance Writers of America, she is knee-deep in revisions for several novels, one of which won the YA category in the 2006 Frontiers in Writing Contest. Another took Honorable Mention in the Romance category in 2008. She is also the owner of An Enchanted Letter™.

Beverly Walker enjoys writing, photography, scrapbooking, and being with her grandchildren. Her stories appear in *Angel Cats Divine Messengers of Comfort*, and several editions of *Chicken Soup for the Soul* books.

Diane Dean White is a freelance writer, columnist and author residing with her husband of thirty-six years on the Carolina Coast. She is the mother of three grown children and three grand-gals. Her stories are embraced by a number of readers and can be found at www.DianeDeanWhite.com.

In 2000, after a teaching career, **Kathryn Wilkens** began to submit essays and articles for publication. Her work has appeared in *Los Angeles Times, Verbatim, Writers' Journal* and other publications. She enjoys traveling and taking photos, then returning to her home in Southern California.

Ferida Wolff is the author of seventeen books for children and two books for adults. Her latest picture book is *The Story Blanket*, co-authored with Harriet May Savitz. Her essays and articles appear in newspapers and magazines. She also writes online for www.grandparents.com and www.seniorwomen.com. Her website is www.feridawolff.com.

Pauline Youd is the author of children's Bible story books, magazine articles, and devotions for both adults and children. Her hobbies include musical comedy theater. Pauline tutors reading and writing, and teaches Sunday school. She lives in California with her husband, Bill, and one very fluffy cat.

Phyllis W. Zeno is a frequent contributor to *Chicken Soup for the Soul* and is the publisher/editor of *Beach Talk* Magazine and Cruise Editor of Ourgenerationflorida.com. She has three children, Richard, Linda and Leslie, eight grandchildren and four great-grandchildren. She recently took her two daughters on a Greek Isle cruise. You can e-mail her at phylliszeno@aol.com.

Chicken Soup for the Soul

Who Is
Jack Canfield?

*J*ack Canfield is the co-creator and editor of the Chicken Soup for the Soul series, which *Time* magazine has called "the publishing phenomenon of the decade." Jack is also the co-author of eight other bestselling books including *The Success Principles™: How to Get from Where You Are to Where You Want to Be*, *Dare to Win*, *The Aladdin Factor*, *You've Got to Read This Book*, and *The Power of Focus: How to Hit Your Business and Personal and Financial Targets with Absolute Certainty*.

Jack is the CEO of the Canfield Training Group in Santa Barbara, California, and founder of the Foundation for Self-Esteem in Culver City, California. He has conducted intensive personal and professional development seminars on the principles of success for over a million people in twenty-three countries. Jack is a dynamic keynote speaker and he has spoken to hundreds of thousands of others at more than 1,000 corporations, universities, professional conferences and conventions, and has been seen by millions more on national television shows such as *The Today Show*, *Fox and Friends*, *Inside Edition*, *Hard Copy*, CNN's *Talk Back Live*, *20/20*, *Eye to Eye*, and the *NBC Nightly News* and the *CBS Evening News*.

Jack is the recipient of many awards and honors, including three honorary doctorates and a Guinness World Records Certificate for having seven books from the *Chicken Soup for the Soul* series appearing on the New York Times bestseller list on May 24, 1998.

You can reach Jack at:

Jack Canfield
The Canfield Companies
P. O. Box 30880 • Santa Barbara, CA 93130
phone: 805-563-2935 • fax: 805-563-2945
www.jackcanfield.com

Who Is
Mark Victor Hansen?

*M*ark Victor Hansen is the co-founder of Chicken Soup for the Soul, along with Jack Canfield. He is also a sought-after keynote speaker, bestselling author, and marketing maven. For more than thirty years, Mark's powerful messages of possibility, opportunity, and action have created powerful change in thousands of organizations and millions of individuals worldwide.

Mark's credentials include a lifetime of entrepreneurial success. He is a prolific writer with many bestselling books, such as *The One Minute Millionaire*, *Cracking the Millionaire Code*, *How to Make the Rest of Your Life the Best of Your Life*, *The Power of Focus*, *The Aladdin Factor*, and *Dare to Win*, in addition to the Chicken Soup for the Soul series. Mark has had a profound influence in the field of human potential through his library of audios, videos, and articles in the areas of big thinking, sales achievement, wealth building, publishing success, and personal and professional development. Mark is also the founder of the MEGA Seminar Series.

He has appeared on *Oprah*, CNN, and *The Today Show*. He has been quoted in *Time*, *U.S. News & World Report*, *USA Today*, *The New York Times*, and *Entrepreneur* and has given countless radio interviews, assuring our planet's people that "You can easily create the life you deserve."

Mark is the recipient of numerous awards that honor his entrepreneurial spirit, philanthropic heart, and business acumen. He is a lifetime member of the Horatio Alger Association of Distinguished Americans, an organization that honored Mark with the prestigious Horatio Alger Award for his extraordinary life achievements.

You can reach Mark at:

Mark Victor Hansen & Associates, Inc.
P. O. Box 7665 • Newport Beach, CA 92658
phone: 949-764-2640 • fax: 949-722-6912
www.markvictorhansen.com

Who Is
D'ette Corona?

*W*hat began for D'ette Corona as a freelancing job in 1999 turned into a full-time job as the Production Coordinator for Chicken Soup for the Soul in 2003. Recently named Assistant Publisher of Chicken Soup for the Soul Publishing, LLC, she is proud to continue to "change the world one story at a time."

Born and raised in California, D'ette received her bachelor of science in business management in 1994. After graduation, she worked for a handful of different companies, but nothing has been as rewarding as her career with Chicken Soup for the Soul.

Chicken Soup for the Soul: My Resolution has been a pleasure to work on for D'ette. After years of reading true life stories, she is still humbled by the heartwarming submissions sent in each and every day—and she is happy to report that she still cries when reading many of them! Her son Bailey is her proudest accomplishment, and her husband George has been her soul mate since they started dating when D'ette was in high school.

Please e-mail D'ette at:
dcorona@chickensoupforthesoul.com

Who Is
Barbara LoMonaco?

*B*arbara LoMonaco has been Editor and Webmaster for Chicken Soup for the Soul since 1998. She grew up in Los Angeles and received her Bachelor of Science degree in Education from the University of Southern California. After graduation she taught at the elementary school level.

Barbara "retired" from teaching when she became pregnant with the first of her three sons and was lucky enough to be able to be a stay-at-home-mom while her boys were growing up. Her sons, John, Michael and Robert, are her proudest accomplishments and she is truly blessed to have two terrific daughters-in-law... Crescent and Christine. Her husband, Frank, has been her soul mate since they started dating when Barbara was in high school. He has always stood beside her and has been her biggest supporter in whatever she has wanted to do.

When the last of her sons left home, Barbara started her job with Chicken Soup for the Soul. Over the many years she has worked there, she has seen, firsthand, how one story or the actions of one person really can make a big difference in someone's life. She feels very blessed to be involved with the Chicken Soup for the Soul organization.

Please e-mail Barbara at:
blomonaco@chickensoupforthesoul.com

Chicken Soup for the Soul

Thank You!

*W*e owe huge thanks to all of our contributors. We know that you pour your hearts and souls into the stories and poems that you share with us, and ultimately with each other. We appreciate your willingness to open up your lives to other Chicken Soup readers.

We can only publish a small percentage of the stories that are submitted, but we read every single one and even the ones that do not appear in the book have an influence on us and on the final manuscript.

A special thank you to Amy Newmark, our Publisher, for conceiving of this book and for her creative vision and expert editing.

We also want to thank Chicken Soup for the Soul Editor Kristiana Glavin for assistance with the final manuscript and proofreading, and Leigh Holmes, who keeps our office running smoothly.

We owe a very special thanks to our Creative Director and book producer, Brian Taylor at Pneuma Books, for his brilliant vision for our covers and interiors. Finally, none of this would be possible without the business and creative leadership of our CEO, Bill Rouhana, and our President, Bob Jacobs.

Chicken Soup for the Soul

Improving Your Life Every Day

Real people sharing real stories—for fifteen years. Now, Chicken Soup for the Soul has gone beyond the bookstore to become a world leader in life improvement. Through books, movies, DVDs, online resources and other partnerships, we bring hope, courage, inspiration and love to hundreds of millions of people around the world. Chicken Soup for the Soul's writers and readers belong to a one-of-a-kind global community, sharing advice, support, guidance, comfort, and knowledge.

Chicken Soup for the Soul stories have been translated into more than forty languages and can be found in more than one hundred countries. Every day, millions of people experience a Chicken Soup for the Soul story in a book, magazine, newspaper or online. As we share our life experiences through these stories, we offer hope, comfort and inspiration to one another. The stories travel from person to person, and from country to country, helping to improve lives everywhere.

Share with Us

e all have had Chicken Soup for the Soul moments in our lives. If you would like to share your story or poem with millions of people around the world, go to www.chickensoup.com and click on "Submit Your Story." You may be able to help another reader, and become a published author at the same time. Some of our past contributors have launched writing and speaking careers from the publication of their stories in our books!

Your stories have the best chance of being used if you submit them through our website, at

www.chickensoup.com

If you do not have access to the Internet, you may submit your stories by mail or by facsimile. Please do not send us any book manuscripts, unless through a literary agent, as these will be automatically discarded.

Chicken Soup for the Soul
P.O. Box 700
Cos Cob, CT 06807-0700
Fax 203-861-7194

Chicken Soup
www.chickensoup.com
for the Soul